THE BROTHERHOOD
OF JOSEPH

A FATHER'S MEMOIR
OF INFERTILITY AND ADOPTION
IN THE 21ST CENTURY

BROOKS HANSEN

MODERN
TIMES

© 2008 by Brooks Hansen

Modern Times is a trademark of Rodale Inc.

Rodale books may be purchased for business or promotional use
or for special sales. For information, please write to:
Special Markets Department, Rodale Inc.,
733 Third Avenue, New York, NY 10017

Printed in the United States of America
Rodale Inc. makes every effort to use acid-free ♾, recycled paper ♻.

Cover design by Joanna Williams
Interior design by Tara Long

Library of Congress Cataloging-in-Publication Data

Hansen, Brooks, date
    The brotherhood of Joseph : a father's memoir of infertility and adoption
in the 21st century / by Brooks Hansen.
        p.   cm.
    ISBN-13 978–1–59486–827–6 hardcover
    ISBN-10 1–59486–827–1 hardcover
    1. Hansen, Brooks, date   2. Adoptive parents—United States—
Biography.   3. Adoption—United States—Psychological aspects.
4. Childlessness—United States—Psychological aspects.   5. Infertility—
United States—Psychological aspects.   6. Fertilization in vitro.   I. Title.
HV874.82.H35A3   2008
362.734′3092—dc22   2008009822

Distributed to the trade by Macmillan

2   4   6   8   10   9   7   5   3   1   hardcover

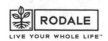

We inspire and enable people to improve their lives and the world around them
For more of our products visit **rodalestore.com** or call 800-848-4735

To Ilya

===

Well, we live by hope.
—J. L. Carr, *A Month in the Country*

CONTENTS

INTRODUCTION

When I first thought about writing this book—an account of my travels in the world of Assisted Reproductive Technology and adoption—the final act had yet to be played. My wife and I were coming off six years of pretty heart-rending frustration, four spent touring all the finest in vitro fertilization clinics in the New York tri-state area, then two more toiling in what seemed like vain, but ever in the hope of adopting a child from somewhere, either the United States or abroad—we were open to either.

In the course of that journey, I can't say we explored absolutely every nook and cranny of those two worlds—the medical and the legal—but for two people of modest means and somewhat involved careers, we definitely covered a lot of ground, and it struck me that, on that account alone, there might be some value in sharing what I'd observed, particularly in the world of reproductive technology. Infertility is as old as the Bible, true, but we have entered a brave new world the past few decades. Thanks to a little scientific ingenuity and, ironically, Western medicine's genius for sterility, the longstanding means of prayer, confusion, and resignation—all swathed in an abiding sense of divine cursedness—have been replaced by an indefinite extension of hope, and a therefore equally indefinite extension of potential failure and despair—again swathed in an abiding sense of divine cursedness. My wife and I never blamed or resented medical technology. It is clearly yielding more happy children and parents who look like each other, but the flip side of such success is that in many cases, it is meting out despair at a rate, and for lengths of time that I'm not sure the human heart was designed for.

This, coupled with the extraordinary challenge posed by adoption these days—the bureaucratic and political webs that encumber the international variety, and the biologically tilted legislation that now places domestic adoptive parents square in the cross-hairs of risk-free exploitation—have created, if you'll pardon the cliché, a "perfect storm" of family-building frustration, all swirling and whirling and thrashing away in a world of famine, neglect, and dire overpopulation.

Adding to the intrigue, and to the reasons compelling this effort, was the fact that I am a man. Women, as we are all now aware, process their experience by expressing it. As a result, though the woman's experience with infertility is no doubt more acute than the man's, it is also generously reflected in the culture at large—in bookstores, the blogosphere, support groups, chat rooms, diaries, letters, and countless private lunches.

I'm not 100 percent sure that men actually do process their experience, but if we do, it isn't by sharing it, and certainly not when the experience in question is as complex, as intimate, and as elusive as this one.

I often, in the midst of our struggles, thought of Joseph the carpenter—earthly and, if you believe the hype, adoptive father of that most famous *in vitro* ever (or more probably just an IUI, come to think of it)—Jesus. Whenever artists portray Joseph in their paintings, they tend to show him asleep, his elbow on his knee, his head in his hand. I guess I always used to think that was because it had been a long night walking from inn to inn; because he'd had a family before, he was tired. And in a certain respect, I probably wasn't so far off. It's no fun pulling the donkey and getting doors slammed in your face. Or building a crib in a manger at three in the morning.

But I've also come to think of Joseph's nap as the artists' way of admitting that they're stumped by this one, this character in the scene: drafted by fate to play his apparently crucial (but clearly not vital) role in this highly improbable event, the consequence of which will demand great sacrifice from him, and which he will offer in faith—to love, to teach his trade, to feed, and fix the roof—to play the perfect supporting part; in other words, to kneel in wonder at the miracle, but not to block the light. Asked to put a face on him, and an expression on his face, artists through the ages could only wonder to themselves, "Who are you, Joseph? Tell us, what does it feel like, to be so much a part and yet to have to stand aside? What have you been thinking? What's going on inside that weary, hoary head of yours?"

. . . Zzzzzzzzzzzzzzzzzzzz.

I can't speak for Joseph. There are some crucial differences between his situation and mine, but the point remains. Just because the male experience of all this sort of thing—of fatherhood not "naturally" come by—is a subtle one, and just because it doesn't often get expressed, that doesn't mean there isn't something worth expressing: what it feels like to be caught up in this blur of plastic cups and paperwork, committed by love, by vow, and by faith in some Divine Order that there is a plan, or if not a plan, then some karmic balance; a hope that ebbs like this must eventually give way to flow; that if ups go down, as everybody knows, then downs must go up, no?

That these tears will be joyful again, and that soon, we'll all see that this is how it was *supposed* to go. On that blind assumption, we proceed, giving ourselves over to a process that otherwise seems completely antithetical to everything we thought we knew about how and what romance begets. We lower our shoulders and muscle through, often quite unpleasantly, trying to figure out how to cope, how to pay, how to laugh, how to change, how to be the man in a situation that simply did not exist in ten thousand years of human history prior to 1981.

I did, however, have misgivings. Though I make my living by writing, I've never been much for confessing in public. Not only do I find something inherently unseemly about it, I just don't think people write about themselves with much authority. Personally I've always preferred the safe confines of a well-told story—true or not—and as I say, I didn't know how this one turned out. Elizabeth and I had completed our "dossier." It was with all the appropriate agencies and ministries, and we had no reason to think that any of these people were crooks or liars (though our instinct in that regard left something to be desired). We were still waiting to find out what happened next, how our story ended, or even *if* it ended. Lacking that, I was, in undertaking a book on these subjects, really just offering my credentials as a smartypants, and it seemed like we have enough of those.

But then we did find out. Not long after I'd started penciling in my first few thoughts and impressions, word came from Russia, and off we went, and what happened next happened next, and what happened next . . . well, I don't want to give anything away, but it would have felt downright stingy not to share it.

So it is in that faith—of wanting to pass along an extraordinary experience—that I present the following, not because I have any advanced degree in the topic or any claim to expertise. I don't. There's nothing here I did not naturally learn along the way, nor, I would submit, are there any recommendations being made, any critiques being levied, agendas being claimed, sides taken, or paths advised. In fact, I shudder to think that anyone would use our experience as any kind of model. All this is is two people's story, from one man's perspective, delivered as honestly as the form allows. Please make no example, nor construe any lessons from it, save for those that are safely inexpressible.

———

Finally, the reader should know that many, but not all, names have been changed, not for the sake of anyone's dignity or reputation, but for the simple reason of privacy. If it were their reputation that concerned me, I'd plaster their names on billboards or rent a plane and sky-write them, for I consider their service to have been so heroic, so professional, so compassionate, and humane. Indeed, I fear that one of the features of our journey that may have been lost in the telling is the extraordinary and very nearly universal generosity of spirit that Elizabeth and I encountered all along the way—from doctors, nurses, technicians, translators, agents, lawyers, concierges, notaries, drivers, judges, social workers, you name it. The only thing more astonishing than the number of people we met and depended upon in helping us toward our goal, is how much they all gave of themselves. I often stood in wonder at the amount of time, care, and attention that these people brought to our problem. Granted, a lot of them were being paid—handsomely. Still, it did not seem possible to me that when we left their offices, or their homes or homelands, that they were going to turn around and apply the same level of focus and energy to the needs of the next couple that walked through their door, to make that couple feel as central to their concerns as we had been made to feel. (When do they write their books? I thought.) But I'm sure they did—not write their books, but wave good-bye to us and open their hearts again to the next forlorn pair who came their way.

So in addition to the silent brotherhood out there who may find comfort in knowing they're not alone, this book is dedicated to all those who helped us, and to all of the remarkable people out there who make it their business to help the childless couple, because the plight of the childless couple—those who want to be parents but cannot seem to find a way—might not seem so extreme in the scheme of things, but I can assure you they are among the saddest and most desperate people on earth, and their hearts are an untapped resource. So to all the people out there who can see that, and try to do something about it, our everlasting thanks and admiration. You are a humbling bunch, and it has been a privilege getting to know you.

PART ONE

INFERTILITY

CHAPTER ONE

THE TROUBLE STARTS

7/20/04

INT. cabin of a plane, 36,000 feet—Night

I am headed back to New York City from California. Elizabeth and I have come back early from our annual West Coast swing to get the last of our paperwork ready for the trip to Russia: Tomsk, Siberia. The far side of the world, where maybe we will meet . . .

. . . Ha ha, very funny. Even as I was writing that—the first sentence of my live account of what we hope will be the end of this long journey—the light above me flickered off.

So let me set the scene, forced by faulty circuitry back to yet another seat. Flying east, we've plunged into night. The lights in the cabin are out. A sparse array of passengers are reading, sleeping, or watching CBS programming. I have shifted seats several times to give Elizabeth more room and to focus on my notes, but also to see if I can find better sound on my headphones. Two and a Half Men *is playing, but lost my attention, so I wondered if the time had come to begin this.*

So I began the very simple, but very daring, sentence that rides the top of the second paragraph there, but as I did, would you believe the reading light above me failed? Blotted my page completely black and stopped my pen; flickered on again to see if I would continue, which I did, and off went the light again. Three times the light did this, and three times I persisted.

Elizabeth noticed from across the aisle. She smiled at the inconvenience, but didn't grasp the irony.

The light came on again, but I had enough. I disentangled myself from the headphones, flung them down, and sassafrassed my way back to the seat behind her, the seat I'm sitting in now, which I presume will let me finish my sentence because I will not be stopped. If this is the seat that lets me finish, then this is the seat I'll sit in, and it has not betrayed me yet. The light, I mean. It has let me write all this, so let me finish, then, before it changes its mind:

My wife Elizabeth and I are headed back to New York City tonight to get the last of our paperwork ready for our trip to Russia:

. . . Tomsk, Siberia.

. . . the far side of the world

. . . where we will finally get to meet our son.

. . . And that, right there in a nutshell, is the story of our last six years.

beth's father taught my father French back in 1951; Elizabeth's mother served as a lay minister, bringing communion to my grandmother. So yes, there are any number of Carpinteria-Babylon scenarios that have Elizabeth and me being unwitting cousins or siblings, which may help explain much of what follows. It also may explain why, even during the years of our hiatus, our minds did wander in the direction of the other from time to time. I always thought of her on her birthday, for instance, which tells you something, since generally speaking I've got a lousy head for dates.

It wasn't until the summer of 1995 that the fates conspired to bring us together again—this time in New York, and once again with the notable and non-too-subtle assistance of our near and dear. Elizabeth had been accepted at a summer-session Shakespearean acting course at the Stella Adler Studios downtown, right next to the Public Theater. Her mother called up my mother to ask if she knew of any free rooms or cheap sublets Elizabeth could use. My mother offered her place. She and my father weren't going to be around much. The apartment was occupied by my younger brother and his roommate fresh out of college—though "fresh" may not be the word.

I was living in a one bedroom (with office) down in the West Village, and took my cue. Vividly I recall the first time I saw her that summer. It was the Fourth of July weekend. My mother had invited her out to Long Island for a couple days before her Shakespeare classes began. I happened to be there as well—with a bunch of friends, a pair of married couples (old friend Nick among them). We were all in the kitchen when she first appeared, entering the back door and setting her duffel on the floor. I took one look at

My wife and I first met when we were teenagers. This was back in 1979. Elizabeth was sixteen. I was fourteen. We met because, though I was born and raised in New York City, large contingents of both my mother's and father's families lived in California. My roots are eucalyptan, so during most of my childhood vacations, my family would go back to a small town just south of Santa Barbara called Carpinteria to see relatives, aunts, uncles, cousins, grandparents.

One summer—we're pretty sure it was 1979—all the parental types had arranged to go off and visit an island off-coast that my grandfather had leased from the Navy, back in the '20s and '30s, to raise sheep. My best friend, Nick, and I were left behind with a gaggle of younger cousins to care for, among them baby twins. Being fourteen, and boys, we weren't quite adequate to the task, so it was wisely decided that an honest-to-God babysitter be brought in, the same girl who usually took care of the twins. This was Elizabeth.

Over the course of those two or three days, she and I developed an apparently mutual infatuation to which neither of us would fess: she being a little older and therefore out of my league; me being a slick New York City kid, and therefore dauntingly sophisticated.

We didn't see each other again for another nineteen years, though we never quite forgot each other either, thanks to the acquaintance of the families. Not only did Elizabeth babysit my cousins, her parents were fixtures and icons at the boarding school that both my father and younger brother attended; Eliza-

her from across the kitchen island and thought to myself, "Damn. There goes my next six weeks."

So Froggy went a-courtin' that summer—a familiar tango of feigned resistance and hot pursuit, all spiced by secrecy: no one must know; they and their prying eyes would only spoil it. That developed into a much less clandestine cross-country romance. Elizabeth was living in San Francisco at the time, teaching. I, a writer unencumbered by external responsibilities, shuttled back and forth between the two cities for another year or so before managing to lasso her back to my little apartment in the Village, sans ring. I am told it was another ten months before I proposed, which at the time didn't seem all that slow to me, though I would later learn there were members of Elizabeth's family who'd all but given up on us, writing off my wife's honest womanhood to my intractable bohemianism (which says more about them than me, trust me).

That was the fall of 1997. We had discovered a small museum up on 107th Street near Riverside Park, a slender brownstone dedicated to the work of a Russian painter/writer/thinker/set designer named Nicholas Roerich. The museum hosted free chamber music recitals on Sunday afternoons, and Riverside Park never looks better than in the fall—all those elm trees with their blondish, jigsawed trunks, the leaves in their resplendent final blush—so we'd decided to stroll along the esplanade above the baseball fields before the concert started. There, on the approximate landing site of a home run I'd hit sixteen years earlier off a lanky Collegiate southpaw named Randy Weiner (and not far from the spot where Elizabeth's father proposed to her mother some forty years before that), I offered my hand. She accepted,

and the point of my story is not to raid the privacy of our courtship any more than I have to. It is simply to say a) that ours was a
union that seemed, as these things go, pretty celestially ordained;
and b) Elizabeth let us bask, oh, I'd say about three minutes in the
glow of our newly forged commitment before hooking my elbow
and starting to schedule, by mutual consent, how soon after the
wedding we would start actually trying to have children.

Her urgency was not without cause. She was thirty-four. I was
thirty-two. So we settled on four months—a carefree season. The
cork landed, and we proceeded to the concert. Schubert. 959.

———

It can't have been too long after that that, I had an interesting
phone conversation with a cousin of mine. He is about ten years
older than me, and I've always enjoyed his company, but for reasons
having mostly to do with age and geography, he is not someone I
ever spent a great deal of time with. He hadn't even meant to call
me, in fact—I just happened to be the one who picked up the phone
that day in the kitchen of my parents' apartment.

He'd heard my big news. He offered his congratulations, then
somewhat out of the blue asked whether we were planning on
having kids. I said yes. He asked how old we were exactly. I told
him, and he said, "Well, get going, because that fertility stuff is
no joke." Something along those lines.

I wouldn't say I felt at all violated by the suggestion, and I
guess I'd had a vague sense that he and his wife had struggled a
while before having their children—two beautiful chips off the
ol' block—but at the time it did strike me as odd that he should be

offering up this fairly intimate bit of advice, given the fact that this conversation probably constituted a good ten percent of our one-on-one time up to that point in our lives, but I said, sure, thanks, I'll tell Mom you called.

In retrospect, I have to commend him both for his prescience and his forthrightness, and many are the times in the years since I've thought about passing along his wisdom. My brother is nine years younger than me, which doesn't make him as young as it used to, but he has been sowing his oats for a while now, and there have been times I wanted to take him aside and tell him, "Don't mess around. If you meet a young woman who lives in a shoe, nab her." I doubt he'd hear it, though, and good for him. Infertility just is one of those things that happens to the other guy, even if he is your brother or your cousin, but my cousin and I have a very simple message, is all I'm saying. There's no point candy-coating it with pat baloney about the Lord's mysterious ways and what was meant to be, or how when it's all behind you it'll feel like it never happened. All that is true enough, I suppose—in a mood— but just as my cousin was there to tell me, I am here to tell you, brother, reader, friend: This fertility thing really *is* no joke. The journey down the road of Western medical ingenuity can fleece you, gut you, pound you, and stunt you. It can worm its way into every corner of your existence, make you feel like you're in a tunnel headed down, and no matter how this book happens to end, there are no promises. For me, the years we spent in all those doctors' offices and clinics was my own personal Viet Nam; a thankless war that lasted far longer than it should have, so staggering, baffling, and punishing that I don't care how much light there is on the other side, nothing will ever make sense of, or remotely justify, what went on inside that tunnel—the length of it, the solitude, the excruciating sense of loss. Nothing will ever give us back the years we spent there, just the two of us clinging to each other, and if I say otherwise, that I'd do it again or it all worked out, or if I so much as mention Nietzsche's name, spank me—I'm a liar. Or shame on me—I just forgot.

———

Anyway, the wedding went great, thanks, and our four months of spontaneity all proceeded according to plan, following which we started "trying"—meaning all that business with the circled dates and thermometers and post-coital headstands. I didn't mind all that much—kind of kinky, in its way. Nor was I particularly concerned that nothing was coming of it. The whole approach seemed so absurd and premeditated, it only stood to reason that we would need some time to make it work.

After about four or five months, though, and still no success, Elizabeth began confessing fears that something might actually be wrong, or at least not right. I still wasn't convinced. I figured we just needed a few more cracks at it—nothing a little Marvin Gaye couldn't fix—but I could sense that her concern might itself be turning into an impediment, so for peace of mind, we scheduled an appointment with a doctor on the Upper West Side, a specialist named Park.

I did not attend, as perhaps in retrospect I should have. According to Elizabeth, Dr. Park glanced at her stats—meaning her date of birth—and advised *in vitro* immediately. Maybe not that bad a call, looking back, but at the time Elizabeth was appalled, and I was too. We weren't going to jump right into the deep end like that. We just wanted a little help, was all. Not *that*. Not yet. So that's the last we saw of Dr. Park, but it was our first official step down the path that would take up the next four years of our lives, leading us through what seemed an endless maze of waiting rooms and doctors' offices, butcher-papered examination tables, plastic plants, pie charts, fishtanks, video fishtanks, "Sample Rooms," counselors' offices, church pews, Lincoln Town Cars, Amtrak platforms, pharmacies, about thirty thousand little vials, thirty thousand shiny needles, and half as many pin-prick bruises, all come and gone like none of it ever happened.

But let me not tax you, or distress myself, with a too-too detailed account of those early years. Suffice to say, and just to orient the novice reader a bit, the Candyland trail of most self-respecting one-bridge-at-a-time child-seeking couples back at the turn of the 21st century snaked its way through the following stops.

1. **Stimulative Drugs**—Generally taken by injection, these are all designed to increase the quantity of eggs produced per cycle (the unassisted norm being one), on the theory that you and your wife are dealing with a finite amount, so best to get them out now while she is relatively young and they're relatively fresh. The degree of stimulation may vary, of course, depending upon drug and dosage, so you can actually spend a long time jiggering around here, trying to find just the right cocktail. Also note: The medical risks of taking such drugs is as yet unclear. The more certain risk is twins, triplets, quadruplets, etc.

2. **Diagnostic Procedures.** If the stimulative drugs don't work. For the men, semen analysis pretty much begins and ends

the diagnostic chapter. There are no surgeries. For women, there are several, all pretty invasive and uncomfortable, from various swabbings and scrapings, to the hysterosalpingogram (HSG), wherein dye is injected into the woman's works, just to see that all the tubes are clear and there aren't any obvious abnormalities. Depending upon the results, further surgeries and/or treatments may follow. Either way, the couple will likely move on to . . .

3. **Intrauterine Insemination (IUI)**—Here, in addition to increasing the dosage and potency of the stimulative drugs, the whole conception process is clinically streamlined—that is, sex itself is eliminated. The male partner plays his part in dim-lit isolation, then lets the doctors in the lab centrifugate his "sample" so as to weed out the lazybones—to winnow your minnows, as it were. The best and brightest are then injected into the woman at the optimal moment, ovulationally speaking.

4. **In Vitro Fertilization (IVF)**—which we will get to, but basically this is where the woman's eggs and the male's sperm are both retrieved separately, then either brought together in a dish, or actually joined via syringe.

5. **Frozen Transfer**—If in the course of an IVF cycle you were left with a surfeit of fertilized eggs, or oocytes, you may try transferring them (i.e., reinserting them in the woman's uterus) at a later date.

6. **Ovum Donation, or Donor Egg**—If it is determined that the wife's eggs are for some reason unusable—or simply not there—the couple may, according to this procedure, retrieve presumably healthy eggs from a third party, or donor, who may be either a stranger chosen by the would-be parents from application

forms ("unknown donor") or a friend or family member ("known donor").

7. **Donor Sperm**—This speaks for itself. Can be "known" or "unknown," obviously, and represents probably the most time-honored practice on the list, going back thousands upon thousands of years, often without the husbands even knowing!

8. **Surrogacy**—Whereby oocytes formed of the mother's eggs and father's sperm are placed in the rented womb of a third party, the "surrogate mother," who is paid to carry the pregnancy to term. Donor eggs and donor sperm may also be used in this procedure.[1]

9. **Adoption**—This requires no medical intervention at all, other than the well-timed bombardment of Valium and amphetamines, and which, as such, isn't really *on* the route, but hovers to the side; a constant, haunting reminder that you're doing all of this to yourself, could stop at any time, turn the board over, and embark upon another path that is—be warned—every bit as expensive and fraught with risk and potential heartbreak.

Obviously, this list gives only a general sense. It is hardly exhaustive and notably fails to include any number of less-Western approaches, many of which can be ventured simultaneously and at the same time as the more aggressive procedures. It should also be said that for each of these steps, countless minor varia-

---

1   As at your local Starbucks, most of these categories are hardly mutually exclusive, meaning that any number of the double-decaf-lowfat-latte permutations do exist, such as the tried and true frozen-cycle-with-the-PGD-donor-sperm-surrogacy route, or as I think it's known on 57th Street, the "Buddy Ebsen."

tions exist, which may or may not apply depending upon the obstacles and resistance of the would-be parents, whose situations, like the situations of all patients everywhere, are ultimately unique. If the husband got his testicles shot off in a laundry incident, for instance, well, then that's easy. Skip to Step 7.

———

In our case, nothing so blessedly obvious presented itself. After a brief round of comparison shopping (involving one memorable visit to a Park Avenue zoo of a practice run by a messianic Norwegian doctor who would months later be indicted for insurance fraud, bless his soul), we settled on an office not too far from the building where I grew up. Clean, well-run, highly touted, and home to what has to be the tawniest, thinnest-hipped clientele this side of Beverly Hills—the sort of people, in other words, who know how to get what they want.

After the usual poking and prodding, our doctor there—a soft-spoken straight-shooter with maybe too much on his plate—was able to identify some potential culprits, but fairly mild stuff as these things go. He set us on the more gradual course we'd been looking for.

We started, as most couples do, with a drug called Clomid, a pill designed to generate multiple eggs per cycle. Pretty simple. It didn't seem to do much good, though, even after we upped the dosage and tinkered with the protocol, so after a few months of that, we added the intrauterine insemination (IUI). That's where I got sent off to the dark room with the La-Z-Boy, but I still can't say as I was too thrown by the experience. There's more than one way to skin a cat, after all, and if IUI was what put us over the top, so be it. Better story.

It didn't, unfortunately, so next we submitted to a few rounds of diagnostic tests. Mine were minor. As I say, all the doctors can really do with the guy is check his sperm. Elizabeth had to endure far more, including the dreaded hysterosalpingogram, but again, nothing particularly decisive was found. Just to dirty up the process a little, we incorporated some of the "alternative" methods into our regime as well, or Elizabeth did: herbal teas, acupuncture, yoga. I ate a lot of pumpkin seeds. I still wasn't too panicked, even when we moved on to the more powerful "stimulative" drugs like Follistim and Gonal-F. That was our first exposure to using needles, and granted, that was a little sobering, but at least we could see we weren't alone. We'd gotten pretty used to the waiting rooms by then, and I'll admit to taking comfort whenever I looked around at the other patients. Our situation may not have been all that rosy, but at least we weren't having to deal with what most of these couples were. That long-faced pair over on the far side of the ficus plant—*Sheesh, what they must be going through. Why, I would never . . .*

I guess you could say I was in a little bit of denial, because it's true—none of what we had done up to that point really felt real to me yet. It all seemed more like a ritual gesture, a way of showing just how determined we were, and obedient, and willing to try anything, but it never felt to me like we were actually addressing the problem. We might as well have been sticking our heads in a lion's mouth, for all I knew. In fact, that's the image that kept coming to mind for me, was a whole row of lions perched on stools, each one bigger and hungrier looking than the last.

There was a day-trip we made down to Southern New Jersey, to a "boutique" mall on the side of the Turnpike. We'd found out about a doctor there who was offering some new approach. Delayed transfer, I think. The ceilings in his office were about seven feet high. The furniture all looked to be about 6' 11", and like it had all been bought at the Liberace estate sale, along with the doctor's hair. He spoke the entire consultation into a hand-held microphone, subjected Elizabeth to a scandalously unnecessary examination, and in the course of our half-hour meeting, tossed at least 500 pages of "literature" into our laps, and that is not an exaggeration—various articles and studies in which he had taken part, all touting his approach. But the clincher was his mentioning an Israeli client of his who'd had to go through *thirteen* IVF cycles before she finally succeeded.

Great, I thought. *My hero.*

Anyway, that's what I mean by a lion's mouth—not just needles and drugs (which I myself didn't really have to suffer), but strange trips to hear strange doctors suggest some slightly different technique than the one we'd been trying, and us nodding our heads like we understood, like that made sense, that might be our answer. I didn't believe it for a second. Doctors don't know everything. And who was to say the problem was even medical? Maybe it was karmic, maybe we were just choking under the pressure—I frankly didn't see how an ice tray could work with that many people watching. But I still went ahead played my part, pried open those jaws and stuck my head all the way in, just to show the lengths we were willing to go to, and just as long as it was understood that this was the last frickin' lion I intended to tempt. That went without saying, each time: no more, fair is fair.

But then the next pregnancy test would come back negative, and we'd find ourselves re-thinking our limits again, wondering if it really made sense to stop at this point, having come this far. Maybe we should just take a little break, because obviously we were hearing all those stories, too, from friends and friends of friends, about how they'd been in the same boat, trying this and trying that and it wasn't until they actually gave up and stopped trying that they got pregnant. Well, thank you, Zenmaster Shitgrin. We tried that, too, not trying, but that didn't seem to work either, so we had to keep going. We had to keep searching, and finally I had to admit that whatever our problem was—biological, psychological, ontological—it definitely had its hooks in us, and it was dragging us, month by month, chair by chair, closer and closer to the dreaded ficus plant and what is by any fair reckoning the essential act of reproductive desperation: in vitro fertilization.

———

I myself was vaguely familiar with the procedure. I think Stone Phillips might have walked me through it a couple times, but I doubt I was paying very close attention—just enough to feel for the plight of the couple on the screen ("poor bastards," as JFK would say). But I suspect it was the compassion that comes with the cold-hearted sidekick, the same one who, when he hears about the lady who got shot on the 178th Street subway platform at two thirty in the morning, thinks to himself, "That's too bad. My heart goes out, but what the hell was she doing on a subway at two thirty in the morning?"

Likewise, whenever I watched those IVF couples on TV, with their trembling chins and interlocked fingers, I'm sure there was a voice somewhere in my head thinking, "Tough break, but that's what you get for trying to have it all." Like it was all Gloria Steinem's fault, like there was some moral to the whole story that I'd be wise enough preemptively to heed.

Well, shut my mouth. I still wasn't sure which "all" it was that Elizabeth and I were trying to have, but after about a year of trying all the less drastic measures, we now found ourselves up on 178th Street at two thirty in the morning, having to decide: subway, or should we call a cab?

The numbers were not encouraging. IVF is an extremely statistics-oriented industry. Most reputable clinics will openly advertise their success rates, set them out on flyers right there next to the *US* magazines, broken down according to all the relevant categories: Male Factor; Female Factor; Women Under 35; Women Over 35; Over 40. Basically, though, one's chances on any given IVF cycle turn out to be not so different from the odds of a "normal" couple—that it, a fertilizationally unchallenged couple (or FUs)—achieving pregnancy in one go after dinner and a bottle of wine: somewhere between 30 and 40 percent.

The problem for me—in addition to the fact that that bottle of wine was going to set us back eighteen thousand dollars—is that I suffer a kind of Calvinist aphasia when it comes to reading odds. You tell me that three out of ten patients have had success in the past, I say, "Great, what's that got to do with me in the future?" It seems to me that everything is either going to happen or it isn't. If it does happen, well, then there was a 100 percent chance of that happening; if it doesn't, then there was apparently zero percent chance of that. And I don't think that makes me a fatalist. You've still got to try, do what you can to make sure the odds turn out to be 100 percent in your favor. Really, I think of myself as more of a post-facto determinist—you know, like when your agent tells you "We all knew that was going to happen." So you tell me IVF works somewhere between 30 and 40 percent of the time, I get it—it means, best case scenario, my chances were about the same as Shaq making his next foul shot (which makes the situation sound pretty dire); or worst case, that Ichiro Suzuki will get a hit on his next at-bat (which for some odd reason makes it seem pretty likely). But what it really meant, to my way of thinking, was that we would probably have to try this at least three times just to figure out if we ever had any chance in the first place.

Now, as that last paragraph indirectly attests, I am a writer, a so-called "literary" novelist who occasionally supplements his income with screenwriting work. At the time, my wife was a teacher of fifth and sixth grade math and drama. Together, we generated a passable income. Heck, if we'd been living in Peoria, we'd have been right up there with the Joneses, but we didn't. We lived in New York City, and as a result led a hand-to-mouth existence. The point being, our life together wasn't really designed to absorb eighteen-thousand-dollar hits casually.

On the other hand, I was raised to believe that the purpose of money is to think about it as little as possible. That means never having too much and never having too little, but it also means *never* letting money be a determining factor in any really important decision or opportunity. You cannot take it with you, after all, and if it should happen that at points along the way that you incur breathtaking heaps of debt in pursuit of a noble goal, well, so be it. Credit cards won the Cold War, didn't they?

The only real question was whether this gamble was pursuant to a noble goal. After all, anyone who can pretend to afford IVF can also probably pretend to afford to adopt, and if you look around and see all the homeless, hungry children in the world, it can seem a little self-important going to such extraordinary lengths just to secure your own puny little genetic legacy.

It can, but here's where I suspect the baby-steps approach might have simplified our decision somewhat; because by the time we'd come to the threshold of IVF, we'd already done so many things we would never have imagined, our minds were pretty well acclimated to the previously unthinkable. All those normative moral and practical considerations had pretty much been swept aside. Money? Who needed money? The politics, the "ethics," what other people thought, even what we ourselves might have thought, or thought we thought at a dinner party five years ago before all this started—none of that mattered anymore. We were on a mission, driven by the same impulse that guides all creatures great and small—humans, frogs, bugs, dogs, and penguins: We wanted to pass down, to propagate, to be vindicated in our choice of mate. Life had thrown an obstacle in our path, fine, but it had also offered us a way around. So what was the question? If you explained to a penguin that his only hope of having a baby penguin would involve test tubes and syringes and plastic cups, granted, he might look at you a little funny, but there's no question in my mind he'd grab the credit card and proceed. And anyone who thinks different— anyone who still clings to the idea that there are ways that God intended and ways He didn't, obviously hasn't heard the one about the reverend and the flood, sacred scripture of all IVF-bound couples:

THE REVEREND AND THE FLOOD

One morning, the Reverend of the church on Main steps outside for a breath of fresh air, and sees there is a flood. The street is a river.

A rowboat comes by, filled with volunteers in raincoats.

"Father, father, climb in. The levees are gone. More rain's coming. Looks like things are only going to get worse."

The Reverend waves his hand. "No, no, don't you worry about me. I have faith. The Lord will provide."

So the boat moves on, and the waters keep rising. In a couple hours, they drive the reverend up into the steeple tower.

A motorboat comes by this time.

"Father, father, grab a line and climb in. The rain's not letting up, but we can get you to dry land."

The Reverend waves them away again. "No, no. I'll be fine. I have faith. The Lord will provide."

Cut to: Another hour later, water yet higher. The Reverend is perched up on top of the steeple. A helicopter swoops down.

"Father, father, grab hold of the ladder! We can still get you out of here."

The reverend still refuses. "No. Thank you, but I'm a

man of faith and I haven't given up yet. The Lord will provide."

So the waters keep rising and lo and behold the Reverend is carried away and drowned.

Up in heaven he appears before God, and he is a little miffed. "Lord," he says, "with all respect, was there some mistake? I was a man of faith. I devoted my life to your service. I trusted you would provide. What just happened there?"

God says, "I'm not sure either. I could have sworn I sent down two boats and a helicopter."

———

So the choice was clear then:

I-CHI-RO! I-CHI-RO! I-CHI-RO! . . .

CHAPTER TWO

IVF, A–Z

So here's how it works—or how it worked, back in our era. The field of reproductive medicine is still so new and aggressive, I'm sure that in the time it takes me to write this, some doctor somewhere will have developed some new way of ironing out a stubborn old wrinkle. Still, if only for purely archival interest:

The first thing you have to do is schedule the procedure, which means meeting with the coordinator at the clinic and getting out your calendars. For the purposes of this example, I am going to suggest that if this meeting takes place in January, the coordinator (most likely a very sympathetic she) may suggest aiming for a transfer date in mid-March, because their office shuts down for two weeks in early April so the doctors can attend conferences. You say fine, mid-March it is. Ides, indeed.

With this in mind, you will now have to go meet with your doctor to decide which protocol—that is, which particular regimen of drugs—you're going to follow. Back in the day there was one called a "flare," whereby your wife would go on the Pill starting in late January, the purpose being to inhibit ovulation so that the doctor can start it up again, with drugs, at a time of his or her choosing.

For even more control of your wife's cycle, however, your doctor is advising against flare in favor of what's called "down reg," which means that, instead, you're going to shut it down with another drug called Lupron.

You agree, because who the hell are you to disagree?

Now, some of you might say, "The husband is who I am," by which you presumably mean Protector and Provider, the one in charge of seeing to it that you and your wife are safe and secure and that you're not getting ripped off—and that's all very noble (if a little retro), don't get me wrong. And if it inclines you to want to roll up your sleeves for the next couple months and take charge of absolutely everything other than your wife's uterus—shopping, cleaning, cooking, driving, bathing, toenail painting—more power to you. And if that sense of responsibility furthermore makes you want to go to the library or get online and turn yourself into the world's foremost uncertified expert on the topic of assisted reproductive technologies, I understand that too. I would only suggest that these kinds of efforts, taken to certain lengths, could just as well be perceived as an aggressive-aggressive overcompensation for the fact that you *are* basically helpless here. This thing really *isn't* happening to you—physically, I mean—and pretending otherwise or getting into some pissing contest with your doctor about the relative virtues of down-reg versus flare might only end up compounding the pressure on what is already a pretty tense situation. Probably the best way to think of your role is as an upbeat functionary, there to help smooth the process as best you can; stay positive without seeming overly excited, calm without seeming like you could care less. It's an admittedly subtle dance. If you're ever having trouble remembering the steps, just think back to your wedding.

In any case, even if you do go online to investigate, I think you'll find that Lupron is an industry standard, and that your doctor is being perfectly reasonable in recommending it. So roundabout the third week of February, you are going to start injecting your wife once a day at the same time of day until further notice. There is a class you must attend—or may already have attended, with other couples—to learn how to do the shots. The nurse demonstrates by using an orange, a grapefruit, or a Nerf football.[2]

There are two kinds of shots you will be called upon to deliver in the course of the cycle: *subcutaneous* and *intramuscular.* Lupron is injected subcutaneously, which basically means *into the fat,* and this is definitely the simpler of the two. It's even possible your wife could administer this injection herself depending upon how squeamish she is, or how obliged you feel to participate in the process in any way you can. Assuming you do feel so obliged, you offer to be the injector. She, for the purposes of quality control, may want to be the one to prepare the shots: swiping down some surface of your kitchen or bathroom with alcohol swabs; cracking the Lupron vials and mixing up the right portions, drawing it into the syringe, screwing on the correct needle, which is very thin and only about an inch long—think of a stylus.

---

2   Be warned, they may also use this class to remind you what you owe them: seven thousand dollars down, with another seven thousand due before retrieval. As for all the drugs and such, that's up to you and your credit cards. You get them yourself, as well as all the syringes, needles, cotton balls, alcohol swabs, and bandages at your local pharmacy.

For a subcutaneous shot, you basically just try to find a good fleshy area—lower belly, maybe, or underside of the upper arm. Keep all comments to yourself, pinch a couple inches, stick in the needle and plunge. The more symmetrical the pinch the better. Otherwise, the needle may go in sideways, or against the grain, and you will cause your wife a burning pain for which she will forgive you, but not really. Once the syringe has been fully discharged, withdraw needle and apply a cotton swab directly to the punctured skin and then Band-Aid the swab in place. Sometimes, there will be a spot of blood. Don't be alarmed.

Do that every day at the same time of day—six thirty p.m., for instance. This either means you will have to be home every day at six thirty, or be willing to pull this maneuver on the fly wherever it is you thought it was so important you had to be—your aunt and uncle's bathroom, the train lavatory, or the ladies' room of the restaurant where you are hosting the big "client dinner."

After about a week of this, your wife will presumably get her period. This is as it should be. She will immediately call the nurse at the clinic, and they will schedule an appointment in two days. You are not obliged to attend this appointment; it's a quickie. Basically they're checking to see that your wife's system is ready to wake up and produce like it's never produced before. Assuming it is, you now start with the stimulative drugs. Again, the cocktail your doctor prescribes may vary—if it's still around, I might suggest Gonal-F, forgotten knight of the round table. The aim is the same: to super-stimulate your wife's ovaries so that they will start producing clusters of eggs.

These shots are a little trickier. These are the *intramuscular* shots. The needle is about two and a half inches long, a much wider gauge, and finding the right spot is no mean feat, because there's really only one area they recommend: high upper-outer quadrant of your wife's buttock, left or right, but not too close to yesterday's shot or the day before, because these can be ouchy. In fact, you might even want to ice down the area beforehand just to numb it. The clinic's recommendation will be to imagine a kind of dial or clock face on the backside of your wife's hip, the idea being to inject around the clock face, alternating sides day to day. It's not bad advice, but not so easy to execute unless you actually use a Magic Marker, which is clearly unworkably demeaning.

But that's not even the really tricky part. The really tricky part is that once you've jammed this longer, thicker needle into the muscle, you have to make sure that you haven't hit veins or capillaries, so you actually have to draw out the syringe just a little bit to see if there's any blood. Assuming there isn't—there very rarely is—then you can proceed with the injection, which is of a much more viscous substance than the Lupron; like a teaspoon of maple syrup.

Again, depending on your technique and how much you've had to drink beforehand, the experience can vary. A good injection is the one she didn't even feel. You're proud when that happens. A bad one she definitely feels, and there'll probably be a little bruise there tomorrow.

So do that twice a day, at twelve-hour intervals. Say, six thirty a.m. and six thirty p.m. And note, just because you have now started the stimulative drugs, that doesn't mean you stop the Lupron. The Lupron shots continue as before—I'm not sure why—but every day at six thirty p.m., about the time the news anchor of your choice is telling you the top stories of the night, you and your wife will be are preparing and administering *two* shots, the Lupron and the stimulant—one into her fat, one into muscle.

Note: This generates a fair amount of garbage, what with all the swabs and paper towels and cracked vials and needles and syringes. Some of this stuff can be thrown away with the rest of your eggshells and coffee grinds. The rest must be collected in an old plastic water bottle for eventual transfer to the hazardous waste bin at your doctor's office. You can expect to fill two half-gallon Poland Spring bottles in the course of your cycle.

———

The most important yield, of course, is eggs. The doctor will begin monitoring their development with increasingly frequent sonograms. He will keep a running count of how many eggs there are, which ovary they're in, and how big they are, because now it's all a timing game. For the cycle we have imagined, aiming at a mid-March Retrieval Day, your wife will probably have to go to the clinic before work on the mornings of March 1, 3, 5, 8, 9, and 10. Something like that.

Again, you will find that you, as husband, don't absolutely have to attend all these appointments. They're early and they're quick. If you're city folk, your wife is cabbing there and then cabbing again straight to work. All you'd really be doing is reading magazines, and there'll be time for that.

As for you, other than the injections, nothing is really required of you until maybe the second or third week of March, at which point you should start to think about rationing your chi in whatever way seems appropriate, depending upon you current rate of release. Experts tell us that for an optimal yield—and I'm speaking here of your sperm count and motility—you might want to take a couple days off before Retrieval Day; that is, if you've been keeping up at all. If not, you might want to start up the engine a week or so before Retrieval, since complete dormancy is also apparently not good for your yield either. Zinc tablets help, and pumpkin seeds are a good source of zinc. Cut down on the alcohol, and needless to say, no more ganja hour in the hot tub. In fact, your wife may, in what will seem an absurdly overly cautious demand, ask you to avoid anything that might overheat your testicles, such as rigorous exercise or wearing briefs. You can try to explain that the scrotum's saving grace is what a brilliant regulator of heat it is, or you may choose to fight another day. Wear boxers and walk around like a cowboy with a hand-fan pointed at your crotch. But not too close.

Over on the egg side of the ledger, you should be starting to see results. The doctor has identified fourteen or fifteen eggs. Eight in the right ovary, six in the left. Not sure about the fifteenth. It could be a cyst. But fourteen is still good and they're developing nicely.

A couple days before the Ides—let's say March 13—your wife should be approaching ovulation time. The calendar says so and at this morning's sonogram, the doctor agrees. The eggs, still fourteen (yep, the fifteenth was a cyst) are nearly ripe, ranging in diameter from 11 to 15 μm, so he schedules the human chorionic gonadotropin (HCG) shot for tonight at ten.

The HCG shot is big. In its way, it is the most crucial of all shots, and therefore must be injected with extreme care. While the Lupron you've been drilling into your wife for the last three weeks or so has been functioning to suppress ovulation, HCG triggers it. HCG ensures the eggs will release in the next forty-eight hours, preferably right around the time that the doctors will be there in their scrubs and masks to retrieve them all.

Given the importance of the shot, you will hire one of the nurses at the clinic to come to your home at the appointed hour to deliver it. Sixty bucks, but worth the peace of mind; that is, unless she is late for some reason. Fifteen minutes. You'll be on the verge of calling her cell when the buzzer sounds. It's snowing. She got caught up in traffic. Some excuse, but you can't help noticing she looks a little decked out for the evening. Black leather jacket. Makeup. There's a bygone day, you think. But she delivers the shot aptly, using a needle which is of a downright vaudevillian length. You pay her sixty dollars, but add ten more because you must give everyone who comes to your door after eight p.m. and who is not your friend an extra ten dollars. She puts her leather jacket back on and leaves for somewhere that is probably a lot of fun. You may take off your pants again and resume watching TV.

Retrieval Day

Oftentimes, your doctor's office and the clinic where the actual IVF procedure is performed are in two different places. Way back when, some of the best clinics in the land were to be found in northern New Jersey. There were a couple there—one in Morristown, one in Livingston. Either one is fine. If you live in the city, it's possible you don't have a car, however, so you may have to schedule the first of what will be several limo rides across state lines. The clinic will help with the arrangements.

At around six thirty a.m. on Saturday morning, a Lincoln Town Car will pull up in front of your building. The driver will call up to let you know he's there, and idle while you get together everything you'll need—water bottle, books, hats, gloves. It snowed a couple days ago because March sucks, so you gingerly you lead your wife down the brownstone steps, even though she's perfectly fine.

As cold as it is outside, it's too hot inside the car. Your wife asks the driver to turn down the heat a little. Having seen the way you helped her down the steps, and knowing that you're headed to some specialty hospital in New Jersey, the driver thinks your wife has cancer, so he kindly obliges. He is very nice. He has family down in Puerto Rico, it turns out.

Not much more than that is said. This is a contemplative drive. You listen to the radio, soft 100, and meditate. As patently ugly as the New Jersey Turnpike is, you realize there's something kind of sublime about it, too. It can yield some pretty epic skies behind all those power lines, belching smokestacks, and low-flying planes. And the landscape actually gets very pretty once you duck into all those old towns. You feel a little like a child sitting there, watching it all slide by, a little bored, a little glazed. It's a familiar sensation, trapped in the back of cars with nothing else to do, forced to think the things you think about things. You realize this is where you did much of your growing up. This is where the little acorn in your head turned into an oak.

Or not.

After about forty-five minutes you pull up to the clinic, festooned with sooty snow drifts. You ask the driver, will he be the one picking you up? He says yes. You think fine, you'll tip him then. Again as if she is an invalid, you guide your wife through the sliding doors, past a makeshift Au Bon Pain in the lobby, and around into the waiting room.

You're not the only ones who took the HCG at ten p.m. Thursday night. There are a half dozen other couples there already, and you're all in the most comfortable clothes you could find. Underneath your parkas and hats, you're dressed a little like it's stockings time on Christmas morning. The mood is just as tense, too, but a little more subdued. The women are performing all the forced rituals of relaxation—thumbing their pulses, their neck and wrists, breathing deep, stroking their bellies, urging their eggs to hold on just a little while longer. Don't want them releasing early, now.

The men are giving off a slightly different energy. Up to this point in the process, the various men in the various waiting rooms have seemed a little off-put by all this, not overtly so, but just a little—like they're not quite sure about the strike the umpire just called. And they look like pretty good hitters, too. Different builds and backgrounds, but there has been a shared determination about their postures. These are men who, when they look in the mirror, see astronauts and gladiators, which shouldn't be all that surprising when you think about it. Anyone willing to lay down eighteen grand on 3-1 odds must have big balls, or think he does. Ironically. So up to now, there has been a kind of low-grade intensity about the men in the room. This morning, however, Game Day, there is an extra calm, even a slight swagger to the way they turn the pages of the sports section, cracking their necks. They're like a bunch of Olympic athletes in the training room.

Because, of course, they've got a job to do today. Finally, a real role to play—and not a half-bad one at that. Indeed, with the possible exception of labor itself, nowhere is the rawness of womankind's deal rendered in starker relief than on Retrieval Day of an IVF cycle. While the wives in here all have the look of deer in headlights, sitting in dreadful expectation of a morning that will combine all the nervous tension of taking the SATs with the surreal invasiveness of the most obscene alien abduction scenarios, their husbands have been called to a duty that is not only famous for taking the edge off, but for which many of them have been practicing literally every day of their life since they were about thirteen.

One by one the names are called. The wives go off to be prepped, put on their open-back nighties and elastic-banded head-caps. The men? Time to show what you're made of, fella. Kiss her good-bye. You wish her good luck. She wishes you the same. You wink, *not a problem*, and follow the nurse off to the Sample Room.

———

Now, if you got all the way to IVF, this probably isn't your first visit to a Sample Room, so you're already somewhat familiar with the work of the interior designer, he with the taste for dim fluorescent lighting, muted blue walls, faux leather chairs and/or couches. The spaces usually aren't large, just enough for the chair; a TV with a VCR, some tapes, and a rack of porno magazines; a sink, liquid soap, a towel dispenser, and usually behind either a door or a partition, a toilet.

So throw in a fridge and you've pretty much got heaven.

Indeed, there's something oddly moving about the no-frills frankness of the furnishings in here, the blunt recognition of who and what they are dealing with. The magazines they've provided—fairly mainstream, airbrushed stuff, may not be to your taste, but still just the idea that someone has thought to leave them there for you, even if it was the guy who just left, is somehow heartwarming. Someone gets you—or is trying to, at any rate.

So if you've done this sort of thing before, then you also probably know that you want to get the clerical stuff out of the way. Fill out the label you'll be sticking on the cup: your name and SSN. Familiarize yourself with the drop-off procedure. Often there is a small cubby in the wall with doors on both sides, for you to leave your cup in when you're done. If the place really has its act together, they will even provide a little light-switch next to the cubby that you can flick on, presumably to illuminate a small red bulb on the other side of the wall, to alert the technicians that there's a pick-up, because there is something a little disconcerting about just leaving your cup in a cubby and walking away. Time is of the essence here, and for all you know, it's just a bunch of monkeys on roller skates over there.

So then set everything up just how you like it. Make sure the door is locked, of course—that is, unless a little risk works for you. Identify what you're willing to touch, what you're not willing to touch. Lay down your various towels and visual aids accordingly. Sometimes these clinics will see fit to provide their own lubricating gel, just for those who need it and really don't think ahead. What's unfortunate is that for some strange reason they leave it out in small vials, standing upright in a rack like tiny, slender milk bottles, which in addition to being kind of visually jarring, is also exceedingly unwieldy and teetery; not a help under the circumstances.

But I don't want to go into too much detail, because I trust you can handle it from here. If you are willing to brave the microbial smorgasbord of the remote control to take a look at the videos they have provided, one caveat: there is a good 30 percent chance that the tape in the monitor is going to feature the work of one Peter North, he being one of the six or seven guys upon whom the mainstream porn industry has relied since I was around eighteen. Mr. North is clean and attractive, very well-equipped, and for the most part, a serviceable pole to hang a pretty flag on—but be warned. Peter North is also the most prodigious ejaculator of his generation. By far. In his prime, the man could caulk the shower stall from the far side of the toilet, which is all well and good for the purposes of recreational entertainment, but when you're locked inside the Sample Room of a fertility clinic in Livingston, New Jersey, pressed to turn in what you are hoping is the most significant performance of your life, watching Peter North do his business can be a little like listening to Horowitz before your fifth-grade piano recital. Perhaps a little more depressing than inspiring.

Anyway, it's the thought that counts, and as I say, if you were born sometime after 1963—that is, in the era of chronic male masturbation—you can probably make do with just about anything. Ruth Buzzi on a tricycle? Why not? So do your things as you see fit. Check the social security number on the label—you really don't want any mix-ups here. Screw on the lid, leave the cup in the cubby, flick the switch, wash up, and make way. Probably you'll be wanting to leave the room pretty quickly once the deed is done, but do check the mirror twice before exiting. Strays have been known to happen, and that can seem a little showy on your return to the waiting room.

———

Or maybe if you've timed it right, you don't even have to go to the waiting room. You can go straight to wherever they've taken your wife and sit with her for a few moments before she heads in for the retrieval, to which you are not invited.

You will return to waiting room to read, take notes, read the paper, whatever passes the time. Maybe nap a little; you've earned it. After about an hour, the surgeon who performed the retrieval will come in and ask to speak to you quietly. She'll tell you how many eggs were retrieved.

Twelve.

"Twelve's not bad."

"No, it's good, and they looked fine. There were two we couldn't get, but she's doing fine. You can go see her now."

The post-op room is partitioned by curtains, behind which all the other hopeful husbands and wives are waiting as well, and coming to. Your wife is still groggy, eating graham crackers and ginger ale.

The nurse comes around to read you your instructions for the next five days or so, what drugs to continue taking, which ones to stop. You should probably pay close attention to this, because your wife isn't retaining much information. You congratulate her anyway: Sounds like she did great.

So now you and your wife return home to wait and rest, recuperate, and keep up with the Tylenol, because when that wears off, she's going to be in some pain; those eggs didn't just pop out on their own. In general you are officially on nurse duty—bringing her everything she wants. Soup. Rice. Dim the lights, rent dumb movies—whatever it takes to pretend to relax, because back at the lab right now, the coats are letting your eggs and sperm have at it. Depending on what you signed on for, the techs have either let the race begin, set them in a dish and left the contestants to their own Darwinian devices; or maybe just to be safe, you signed on for ICSII (an extra three thousand dollars), meaning a doctor has personally selected what strikes him or her as being the most sprightly spermatozoa in your sample, and has actually injected them into the waiting eggs.

And what possible difference could that make?

The call comes at around five o'clock the following day.

"Looks like we've got ten."

Ten. Meaning that of the twelve eggs retrieved, ten have fertilized. Again, not bad. Pretty good, in fact. You tell your wife. She smiles, but this afternoon's Tylenol is wearing off. If you're lucky, maybe you find an old Nick and Nora movie, keep the volume down, lights low, let the day pass, say prayers for the ten little Indians down in New Jersey . . .

You will keep doing this for the next few days, keeping your fingers crossed, visiting church pews or skating rinks or wherever you like to go to direct all the positive energy, but New Jersey is still where the real action is. That's where the battle is being waged, and even now some of the troops are probably falling by the wayside. Who knows why? Chromosomal abnnormality. Doc picked a dud. Lack of zest. Maybe they just felt the whole thing was a little contrived.

But you're hoping as many as possible can hang in there, because in less than a week's time, the survivors will be transferred back into your wife's womb, which means her recovery is paramount. She should take a day or two off because she's still feeling sore. She's on mild painkillers and antibiotics. And you should probably put your work on the back burner. Maybe check in once or twice just for the sake of normalcy.

Roundabout Thursday the call comes.

"Five."

Five have survived. Three look good. They're "fours and fives." (The doctors are giving them grades already.) The other two, we'll see. In any case, they've scheduled you for transfer on Friday.

So five made it. Five's not bad. Your wife agrees. Five would be too many, if it all worked out.

Transfer Day

Transfer Day is a lot like Retrieval Day, itinerarily speaking, but easier. You don't have to wake up so early. All transfers happen in the afternoon, and you, the husband, have nothing to do really, other than to offer moral support.

The Town Car comes to pick you up at about eleven a.m. Same driver drives you out. The snow has more or less melted now. You look at the sky and the power lines, the planes, and later, the pretty houses. You ponder your life in silence. You hold hands intermittently.

The waiting room at the clinic is filled with much the same cast of characters, the women all looking a little less nervous; the men, a little less cocky. Again, you all go in order, but this time you accompany your wife the whole way through. You're there when she changes into her little string-tie gown and sanitary slippers. Together you wait in the pre-op room with all the other couples, but all partitioned from one another by curtains on rails. You get a rolling bed, a chair, a small closet. They also give you some doctor clothes to wear, which is always fun. Your wife admires the look. This is what you'd look like if you were a surgeon, or if you just played one on TV.

You can hear outside, the real surgeon has arrived, and he's making his opening rounds, going from couple to couple and telling them one by one how many of their eggs have survived; how many they'll be transferring today. You try not to listen. Your wife drinks her bottled water—it's important her bladder be full for the procedure. You thumb through magazines. Damn that Reese Witherspoon and Ryan Phillippe—some people just have all the luck. But Reese complains of having an average body, and you're inclined to believe it, actually.

Finally the doctor gets to your partition and tells you. Two. Two eggs have made it. You sink a little. You'd been hoping for three at least. Three is a magic number.

But they look good, he says. They're "fives" apparently, so that's good. He has brought you a photograph of them, and they do look good for a pair of five-celled wee bairns. One is a little less symmetrical, but you tell yourself you love them equally.

So now you sit and wait some more for your turn. You scoot your chair up to the bed and keep your wife's feet warm, as one by one, the couples ahead of you are rolled in and then out of the operating room. These things don't take very long. About ten minutes each.

You study the curtain. A part of the pattern, there amidst the harmless swirls and stars, is the recurring image of a game of tic-tac-toe, and as you look at it, you realize what's so odd is that someone has actually won. The 'x' player has completed a diagonal column, and swiped it with a line.

So who was the jackass playing the 'o's?, you wonder.

And now you hear the couple ahead of you is finished. There's a tap on the curtain. The nurse and the doctor both come in to wheel your wife into the operating room. You follow in your blue scrubs and paper slippers. You put on your face mask as well.

It's dark inside, and calm, and there's a large suspended monitor. Music is playing—Enya. There is another doctor back behind a glass partition, like an engineer in a recording studio, and you can see on the monitor that she's sucking the two little oocytes into a tube, and handing them over to the doctor, and it goes on from there. You hold your wife's hand. This could be it. These could be the ones. This is the closest you've ever gotten, and you can watch the whole thing live on a monitor, the long, slender tube entering your wife's uterus, the oocytes popping out the end and settling in place, all to the tune of "Orinoco Flow."

Once they're done you help wheel her back out into the light of the pre-op room, back to the safety and comfort of your curtained partition, for one more round of waiting.

The attending nurse enters briefly to go over your instructions for the next few days. What meds to take. No rigorous exercise. No swimming. You both nod.

Your wife asks, "But how do we know they won't slip out, even now? I mean, I think I might have just felt something." The nurse is reassuring. She has had to answer this question five times already this morning. "They won't slip out. Think of it as being like a peanut butter sandwich down there."

You think to yourself, not only is that kind of gross, it's also not very reassuring. Things fall out of peanut butter sandwiches all the time.

The nurse says she has called your driver already. He'll be here in ten minutes, so you try to relax, though your wife really has to pee now. You re-contemplate the tic-tac-toe game on the curtain, try to reconstruct the sequence of moves—what ingenious plan was Mr. 'o' hatching that so completely distracted him from what 'x' was up to? Then you see that in the very next move, no matter what 'o' did, 'x' was on the verge of completing *another* line.

So not only did this 'o' guy actually lose at tic-tac-toe, he got his ass kicked.

You show your wife. "Maybe he should run for President."

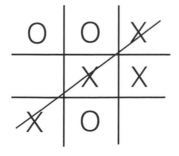

The room is quiet and, well, in a word—pregnant. Your heart goes out to everyone in it, and theirs to you. You wish them well as couple by couple they pad out the door, wives on husbands' arms. All in this together.

After about twenty minutes, the attending nurse taps your curtain again. Time to go. Did your wife want to go to the bathroom?

Yes. They lead her off. You start gathering together your things, remove your scrubs; grab coats, hats, forms, and oocyte photos. And a sandwich is actually starting to sound pretty good. You make a pit stop at the Au Bon Pain on the way out.

———

It'll be two weeks before you know for sure. In the meantime, you'll try to resume your life. After a couple days, your wife goes back to work. You go back to work.

You will have been instructed not to read much into anything your wife may be feeling in the way of symptoms. They say the effects of oncoming menses and pregnancy can be very similar, depending upon the woman. But the two of you are pretty familiar with your wife's cycle; the sorts of headaches, cramps, the scent, and it's difficult to get out of your mind the slow but sure attrition of candidates you've been monitoring since early in the month: from the fifteen eggs in her ovaries, to the twelve they got out, then the ten that fertilized, the five that survived, the two that made it to transfer day . . .

And your wife says she has begun to spot. The nurses on the phone say that's perfectly normal, but your wife also got one of those headaches today, and when you kiss her tummy good night tonight, you want to feel like there's something in there, one or two little candles, but you don't, and you don't know what it would feel like if you did.

———

April 1, ironically. The call to confirm comes late in the afternoon. The bad news always waits, and your pretty sure your wife's period began in earnest this morning. She didn't say, but you saw the wrapper in the basket in the bathroom.

The nurse's voice is filled with authentic regret. "I'm sorry," and she means it, and you say, "Thanks." You're not really sure what to say. You hang up the phone and wander off toward the bed—well, it depends on whether the call came when you were alone. If your wife is out buying groceries but you stayed home just to be sure someone would be there if the nurse did call, then you stagger off to your bed and start weeping; or if your wife is there, you nod at her, yes, they said no, and you both pretend to continue doing what you were doing when the phone rang; fold the laundry, put away the dishes. Then a little later the two of you go back to your bed and you weep together.

CHAPTER THREE

THE TOLL

Now just exactly how many times Elizabeth and I put ourselves through the process just described, it's hard to say. Given all the minor variations that can be thrown in along the way, freezing things and trying again later, the numbers get a little fuzzy. But it was a lot, enough that this is where our story becomes more cautionary than typical.

But our reasons were sound, I tell you. As I say, none of the diagnostic procedures the doctors ran ever turned up anything that IVF wasn't specifically designed to address, and our numbers for each cycle—the various indices by which you might measure a couple's chances—were actually pretty good. Really, the only thing that ever discouraged the next attempt was the failure of the last, which the doctors all made clear. None of the men or women we dealt with was ever remotely deceptive or coercive. Still, to me it just felt like we were that solid .280 hitter who happens to go hitless for the weekend: A couple line drives into the third baseman's glove; umpire makes a rotten call; circus catch in right field and before you know it, you're 0 for your last 10. But that's no reason to panic. Willie Mays started his career 0 for 13.

It also probably didn't help that I am saddled with a very stick-to-the-plan mentality. When I was a kid, I never really liked those old Roadrunner cartoons; it used to frustrate me so much having to watch the coyote put all that effort into his ingenious schemes only to abandon them after the first try. I always wanted to shout at the screen, "No! Do that one again! It'll work, I swear."

Also, there is the fact that Elizabeth did get pregnant—once, on our third IVF. For about two months one autumn, we were permitted to think that all those needles and car trips had worked. We told no one except closest family, and otherwise floated in a kind of two-person anesthetic cloud, moving gingerly, looking over our shoulders like the couple who realizes they never got billed for dessert.

Eight weeks in, reality caught up. My two-year lease down in the Village had finally expired (after twelve years), so Elizabeth and I spent a very stupid day apartment hunting. We got caught in a cold raw rain on the Upper East Side, kept pressing on, walking way too much, hiding out from the wind in building entrances, pushing on, finding nothing. The next day Elizabeth called me from the doctor's office. She'd gone for an ultrasound, and the doctor said he couldn't find the heartbeat. I cabbed up and met her at another office, an unfamiliar one also on the Upper East Side. The waiting room was intensely crowded, and for some karmically fercocked reason, the publicist for the paperback of my latest book was there as well, waiting for something presumably less upsetting. She was over to my left, trying to pretend she hadn't seen me, Elizabeth was beside me, stunned and grieving;

I was in my chair, feeling all that sweet relief dissolving like the sugar castle I'd deep down known it was.

The D&C revealed the embryo to be chromosomally sound, which was good news and bad. That meant, had the fetus developed to term, there was no reason to think it wouldn't have been a healthy baby. No reason not to try again, in other words, and, well, anyone who has ever played a slot machine will understand: if it took you three cranks to come up triple cherries, but then something went unaccountably wrong—fire in the casino, tiger on the loose—you are probably, if you are of a determined mind, going to give yourself three more cranks at it as soon as all the smoke has cleared, because maybe that's just the way you work. Maybe that's your rate. That's what it takes for you.

And if on the last try, the third try of your second round, something weird happened again, like the doctor who was supposed to be monitoring your case happened not to be in the office when a crucial decision had to be made about the timing of the HCG shot, and if another doctor you didn't really know made what seemed like an odd call based upon your history, and if you think that might have contributed to a botched cycle, well, you are probably going to have to give it an*other* try, aren't you? Just to be sure, just to be satisfied that you gave it your best.

And by the time you're done with all those, who knows? Maybe by then there's some new technique someone somewhere came up with. Or maybe insurance has decided to kick in on more of these procedures. Maybe by the time you've endured all that, your hearts and minds are so scarred and numb, so adept at wrapping themselves around heretofore unthinkable options, you're ready to move on to some of the more creative permutations they have to offer.

You get the picture. A stubborn man and wife can really lose their lives to this stuff if they're not careful, and Elizabeth and I were a pair of mules, as it turned out. At the office we went to, they kept file folders for all the patients, with test results and records of previous cycles. The nurses literally staggered beneath ours when they pulled it down, a giant spilling heap of failures past, testifying to the fact that the months were now turning into years, the years were turning into whole new years, new presidential administrations, new Olympic champions, and there we were, still thumbing through magazines, signing in, plugging away with our needles and Band-Aids, and not because we were stupid or insane or suckers. It was just because we wanted this thing so damn much. We were desperate, and each time we failed, we only got more desperate.

It was—if you'll pardon the diminishing comparison—a little like waiting for a taxi in the rain when you're already late for that appointment. You wait and you wait, and the longer you wait, the longer you're going to wait because you know the second you give up and take the bus instead, a whole fleet of empty cabs is going to come pouring down the street and pass you in your window seat like a gang of mooning high-schoolers.

It's like that, except the appointment you're missing is your life as you'd been picturing it.

———

And that was the real tragedy. It's one thing not to get what you want. The loss of a dream— especially if that dream is progeny— hurts. But it was only ever a dream, and I hate to say it, but over time I actually got used to the disappointment. I felt like I was the one consoling the nurses, telling them they'd done everything they could.

But what's worse than losing something that never was is the loss of what's happening right now. This seemingly endless cycle of expenditure, effort, hope, and heartbreak was eating up years we couldn't have back, but we were helpless to stop it. One way or another, we had to fix this problem. We had to become a family, and until we were, everything else would have to wait.

And that's probably the one thing about infertility that people on the outside don't quite get, the one thing I'd want to convey to friends and family—because after a while we did begin to sense their impatience, a silent tipping point at which their compassion turned into irritation at having to whisper every time someone *else* got pregnant, or had good news. We could hear the whispers, too, and believe me, no one wanted to move on more than we did, but the problem with infertility in the 21st century is you can't. It's not like getting a limb shot off, with all respect, or having your house burn down—where some horrible event occurs that will change your life forever, but at least it only happens once. At least you're forced to adjust, to adapt to the fact that there is no hope, it's not coming back. With infertility there's always hope. There's always some new doctor out there offering some new twist, so you are constantly having to decide—should we, shouldn't we? Third time's a charm, or maybe flare this time. Or donor egg. Or surrogacy. And whatever you decide, you better decide fast, like right now while the wound is still fresh and oozing, because time's a-wasting. The longer you wait, the slimmer your chances are going to be. Those eggs aren't getting any fresher. . . .

That's the real horror of it, how unrelenting the process is, and even now I'm not prepared to assess the quality of the decisions Elizabeth and I made. Fate can revise with a flick of the wrist. All I know is that for around four years running, Elizabeth and I were either a) preparing for the upcoming cycle with the twice-daily shots and late-night runs to the drugstore; b) actually in the midst of the cycle itself, meaning all those car trips to New Jersey for the retrievals and the transfers and the authorized pregnancy tests; or c) drying our eyes, dusting ourselves off, and trying to figure out what the next step was going to be. Truly, not a second passed that did not find us in one of those three godawful places. Everything else was wallpaper, a way of biding time for now, and averting our eyes from all the damage this was doing— and the damage was considerable.

———

The financial hit was certainly the least important in the scheme of things, but probably should not go without saying. All our savings were devoured, every IRA and piggy bank was busted and emptied. Those mutual funds that got clobbered in the "correction" of 2000, I'm afraid they didn't have time to claw their way back to principal. We swallowed the loss and cleared them out too. Had to. Credit cards? I can't say as they were maxed—today's usury industry is far too smart and unfettered for that—but the balances were jaw-dropping, and teetering at rates that would make John Gotti blush. Every cent we made got swallowed up like crumbs feeding a beast. Often as not, rent got paid by those checks you get in the mail from your credit card company and immediately throw away; those, or mad dashes to the bank for cash advances, or wired money from relatives or producers who owe you for that re-upped option. It was ugly. Financially, we were digging ourselves a hole that made college loans look like that drink you owe your high school buddy. And not a penny had gone toward building anything. We weren't one step closer to having kids than we were when we started. It was pure, down-the-toilet, loss.

Our social life didn't fare much better. A lot of our closest friends were having children, and that was hard. We hung in there at those downtown brunches, nursing our mimosas while they all traded wallet photos and tips on car seats, but when the front door opened again and another line of strollers rattled in bearing balloons and painted faces, it got to be a bit much. We ducked out quietly, vowing to ourselves that it wasn't always going to be this way. Someday we'd be ourselves again, not these dull stand-ins with glazed eyes and wan smiles.

Not that it was just our breeding friends we felt like we were shortchanging. It was the gays, too, and the bachelors, the gay bachelors, the widows, spinsters, dogs, cats. Basically all our exchanges felt as if they'd been wrapped in a gauze of bland inauthenticity, where the one thing worth talking about was the one thing I couldn't.

And you may be thinking, "Why not? Isn't that what friendship is for? Being there for each other when the going gets tough?" In most situations, I'd agree, but again, infertility if pretty ingeniously rigged. It really is like a disease, not just because of all the hospital stays, and bills, and drugs, and side-effects, etcetera—but because once you've been diagnosed, you quickly come to find the only people you can really talk to about it are the ones who've been through it too—them and family. Otherwise, it's just too draining having to explain it all, or account for your decision, because if these people really do love you and care about you, they're going to want to help. They're going to want to know how things are going, how many eggs, when's the retrieval? What can they do? Bring soup? What kind? Worse, they may even have opinions, a cousin who's been through the same thing and knows a doctor outside Philadelphia. And when you're right in the middle of one of these procedures—as we always were—all that interest and advice just turns into static, no matter how well intended. It saps the energy you need to succeed, and if you engage it too much, pretty soon you find that you're not just the principal subjects and executors of this completely surreal procedure, you have become its press spokesman as well; meaning, if you're wife *doesn't* get pregnant—if for some strange reason 70 percent defeats 30 percent again—not only will you have to deal with your own heartbreak and disappointment, you will have to bear the burden of everyone else's as well, for you. I suppose for some people, this may be consoling. For me, no. For me, better to wait, because don't forget, there could be good news too. This all might work out— soon, I swear—so why not wait until you can surprise everyone with a bottle of champagne.

———

The problem, of course, was that "soon" kept getting pushed back and back, and as I say, that's what eventually took its toll. On us,

Elizabeth and me. Because back at the beginning of our run, we weren't actually doing that badly. Infertility represented such a direct assault on our whole reason for being—married—there were respects in which it kind of steeled us, the same way a good team comes together when their star player blows out his knee in the first quarter. We weren't going to let that beat us. We hunkered down. We played better 'd.' Passed the ball. We figured out what our roles were and we performed them. If you'd seen us with those syringes, you'd know what I was talking about. We didn't point fingers. We didn't undermine. Whatever tectonic shifts had taken place beneath the bedroom or the kitchen—the latent sense of entitlement and blame, and all the unspoken compensations that might derive from there—we ignored. The way I saw it, the fact that we had chosen to be together was far more significant— diagnostically speaking, I mean—than sperm counts or endometriosis or motility or FSH levels. If there was dysfunction here, it happened the moment we sighted each other as potential mates, and it was a moment we both willingly participated in, so let's just do what we need to do.

I'm not pretending we were saints or that any part of it was easy. Neighbors definitely got awakened along the way, and many a paint chip fell from the shuddering door jamb. I'm simply saying that—at the beginning at least—our experience only served to make plain what marriage is anyway: two people deciding to team up, in full and solemn recognition of the fact that at points along the way, they are probably going to find themselves in some tough spots. They're going to feel like they're lost at sea sometimes, or stuck in a trench. That's what happened to us. We hadn't expected to be thrown in there so soon, or to have to stay for so long, but we were all we had, and that's how it was going to be until we figured out a way to clear this thing.

Ah, but there's that word again, *until*. *Until until until*. You can get into trouble with that word. Or the phrase *Just for now*. *We'll do it this way, just for now, until this passes*. That approach may work for three months, or six, but a year? Two years? A team can do the right things for only so long before the weaknesses start to show, and Elizabeth and I were under no illusion. We weren't all that well designed to be a couple without a child. So the question was, at what point did all that good behavior become a mask, or begin to ransom the rest of our relationship—make it so that nothing else ever got discussed or ironed out, for fear it might betray some deeper resentment, or prey upon a known weakness? At what point did the sense of responsibility we felt toward each other ignore the fact that we were different people? We'd come into this experience from different perspectives; obviously it was affecting us differently. We were changing. Or at least I was. The person I was becoming was not the person I'd been, and so far as I could tell, the change was not for the better.

———

Up until this whole fertility debacle, I'd always thought of myself as being pretty successful. No rags-to-riches hero, by any stretch, but someone who'd played his fortunes well, knew how to sight some pretty ambitious goals and see them through. So this prolonged ordeal with the clinics and syringes wasn't just painful and discouraging; it pretty much defied everything I thought I knew about myself. And as I say, I don't think I was the only man in those waiting rooms who felt that way. Yet for most of my fellow astronauts and gunslingers, their little excursion down into northern New Jersey turned out to be just one more illustration of how badass they really were. They hit a snag, studied up, found the best clinic on earth, got good with a syringe and—boom— problem solved. "I'd like you to meet my triplets, Zooey, Joey, and Chloe."

Me? Four years into this with nothing to show for it but debt that I had no business incurring, I honestly didn't know what was going on, except that my life seemed to be passing me by. The opportunities I might have taken, places I might have gone, challenges I might have tried, I simply couldn't. I was too broke, too confined by the process, too busy doing the one thing that all successful people understand you are not supposed to do: waiting; waiting for the gift that wouldn't come; living in the presence of the unyielding absence.

A better man might have found better ways to make his feelings known. I chose a more typical route, "acting out" in one way or another—you'll just have to use your imagination—but when Elizabeth called me on it, I'd use the ensuing dust-up as an opportunity to say what I was really feeling. It was the old "Well, how do you expect me to act?" routine, complete with choreography, where the woman keeps retreating behind closed doors and the man keeps pursuing, just to finish what he has to say because if he doesn't say it now at the top of his lungs, he's never going to say it at all. The kind of scenes that make you glad you're not a celebrity.

One of our doozies dragged us out onto Riverside Drive one night. It was spring, I think, and I was hounding her, trying to make my point, and in my head, what I meant to express wasn't so bad. Kind of nice, if you think about it. All I wanted her to know was that she shouldn't be feeling guilty about the whole genetic legacy thing—I honestly didn't care anymore. Frankly, at that point, if she had gotten pregnant, I'd have been pissed at the kid for taking so long. What was killing me was what this was doing to our lives here and now, trapping us, putting everything on hold like this, and eating up years we couldn't have back, like I said.

I'm guessing that's not how it came out, though, or maybe it did, but the only answer I got came from a loud male voice, seven stories above us.

"Leave her alone!"

That shut me up. I was torn between wanting to run up to that guy's apartment and shove a mailbox up his ass for not minding his own business, or just crawling down a storm drain because he was right. I should have left her alone, or at least stopped punishing her for the fact that I felt helpless here, for the first time in my life. I'd always thought of myself as being someone who knows how to get things—a lucky fella with smarts to boot—but here I'd had my first bout with real adversity, and it was mopping the floor with me.

———

One question was, How personally should I be taking all this? Was this some kind of payback for my prior good fortune? Was this a test? Or was there no sense to be made? Was meaning really just a mirage, and I, a happy little bug who happened to get caught on the wrong breeze and wound up a smudge on a windshield? It happens.

Well, something else you should probably know about me is that I was raised Catholic, so that particular brand of nihilism—the sweet release of thinking *Nothing matters, so don't beat yourself up*—wasn't really an option. If you're raised in as stout-hearted a faith as Catholicism, you can lapse for as long as you want, you can revise your personal creed to your heart's content—but I still don't think there's any way to entirely shed the sense that when you think, Someone is listening; that your thoughts and actions are all being registered somewhere, and if not answered, then certainly absorbed and processed; that life, as such, really never stops being a prayer to the Almighty, just a very sloppy one that devolves into lengthy passages of dither, solipsism, and profanity. The point is, if Someone is listening—if there's some transaction taking place between your little mind and the greater Mind of the Cosmos—well, then surely there is Meaning. It's simply a question of whether you can figure out what that Meaning is.

In this instance, it didn't seem like it should be so hard. The whole thing was so ironic, for one: that I—me, of all people, who had always seemed to be so gifted—should be denied the one gift that is by all accounts the greatest of all, and which also happens to be the most democratically distributed, the one that every asshole and his brother seems to get for neglecting to wear a condom, I couldn't have despite the efforts of all the King's horses and all the King's men. There was definitely *some* sense to be made here.

And yet, while in the past I'd always felt that my Creator and I had enjoyed a fairly lucid exchange, I now felt like I was having a conversation with the PA system at the 14th Street subway station. I had no idea what was being communicated to me, or why, even though I'd never tried so hard to listen. Which was probably the problem.

Some of this listening took place in church. Typically, Elizabeth and I did find ourselves returning to the pew more often now in our hour of need, but our prayers weren't silly little prayers of petition: *Please help me out, I promise I'll be better.* All we really ever asked for was some clue, or the strength, or the clarity of vision to know what we *should* do, where to put our energy, what to pray *for.* For somewhat the same reason we also consulted psychic types, and reflexologists and anyone else we thought might be able to point us in the right direction, and it wasn't a complete waste of time, either, psychics being a relatively cheap way of finding out what you want to hear.

I will say that Elizabeth was the one who tended to pursue these more trodden paths. My own efforts weren't quite so MOR, but were no less maudlin. Skating in the park one autumn day, asking for a sign, I was struck in the face by a leaf. I kept the leaf in my leather satchel for the next two years. Or another time, during a phone conversation at my desk, the inadvertent scribbling of my pen revealed the unmistakable profile of a baby. I tore the image from the corner of my notebook and taped it to the inside of my drawer.

Why? What for? I don't know. Just searching, I guess. Hoping. Trying to make some sense, and though it's always a little suspect, organizing your experience in retrospect like this, I think it's fair to say that my outlook tended to alternate between two closely related but rival interpretations of what was going on, and which of them held sway any given moment depended upon how much, or how recently, I'd eaten.

On the one hand, there was a part of me—the better-fed part—that was perfectly capable of regarding the whole experience as an apparently necessary expression of the Universal Will; an upsetting one, no question—I didn't want to deny the feelings that our struggles seemed designed to elicit—but at the same time I didn't want to take them too personally. Better to treat them as something that apparently needed to happen—a dramatization, if you will, of feelings that I, Brooks Hansen, in my role as proxy for a certain set of experiences and emotions that the Universal Mind was, for whatever reason, interested in exploring, had been called upon to endure, to exercise, and presumably at some point to transcend, which in the deepest recesses of my being I trusted I would be able to do. I mean, *come on*. We weren't the first couple to run into this kind of trouble, and I figured if I hadn't garnered enough resources along the way to cope with a little misfortune, then I deserved my pain. Again, in the deep, well-fed place, I assumed that I would be handling this in the same way that the healthy-minded soul handles anything: that is, in recognition of the fact that, in the first place, the realm in which this whole drama was being played—i.e. the so-called "real world"—really wasn't anything of the kind, was at best a substanceless reflection of the Truth, and at worst a gross distortion. One probably shouldn't take too much stock in the harvest of this realm, therefore, since—in the second place—the only real gift any of us is given is the Present Moment, and the only thing of value to be found there is in the use of one thing to another. Service. That is as much as any of us are given to know of the Divine, so what did it matter who got what or why? Simply love, be of service, and let the rest happen through you, as the sky allows a cloud to pass.

Just don't bogart that joint, dude.

Find me six or seven hours removed from my last good meal, feeling a little more hollow and peckish, I'll admit it was hard not to take this line of thinking one step farther and wonder if the Universe's dramatic impulse here might not be a little more motivated than I was giving it credit for. Perhaps the reason it had chosen *me* to feel this way was because it had detected some flaw in the player—something rotten at the core—and was offering a direct response. No more of this. That's what they say about miscarriages, isn't it? Nature's way . . .

Sounds absurd, I know—a grown man thinking like that. We know better. Life is strewn with so much injustice, so much senseless tragedy, the notion that what happens is any reflection of one's worth or karmic due, why it's practically pagan. At the very least it's narcissistic. And particularly if we're talking about who gets to have children—of all the institutions that we may safely conclude are not meritocracies, I think parenthood would have to be at the top of the list.

Still, when it's you, when you're the one with your nose pressed up against life's window, it's hard not to catch sight of the reflection and wonder if you're not somehow to blame. Particularly these days, with all the Clomid and the Lupron and spermal centrifuges, if you and your wife can't manage to squeeze out one measly hatchling, you've got to wonder, Did I do something? Is what I get for . . . marrying an acorn from the next tree down? Choosing a woman who seemed like she'd make such a good mother? For being that calculating? Or was it something worse?

I once broached this subject with a counselor Elizabeth and I were seeing—the idea that our troubles might reflect a measure of accountability. I hadn't gotten the last syllable out of my mouth—for all she knew, I was simply suggesting that God had decided to "pun" me—but she practically leapt out of her chair. "No, you can't think that!"

And of course I knew what she meant: She meant that I was only going to make things harder on myself, compound my burden, if I started blaming myself. But how could I *not*? Man has always taken responsibility for the things that happen to him, from being hit with the latest plague to having his clothes thrown out his girlfriend's window. We like to think we know why something is happening and whether we are to blame, and while it's all well and good to act as if we've refined our sense of what we can and cannot influence—that somehow a few Russian novelists and French philosophers woke us up from the vanity of thinking that morality and consequence were anything but markers of our own device—it is also the case that we live in a culture that embraces the concept of holistic karma like never before. The notion of outright "punishment" may be a little fire-and-brimstone for someone educated in the Northeastern Corridor, but it's not as if those red-faced Baptists and Evangelicals are the only ones out there selling the notion of universal accountability. It's the most self-proclaimedly evolved gurus living in and around the Bay Area and Seattle, too—and even I, by certain perfectly commendable readings—who promote the idea that we are the creators of our reality, including the moon and stars, two-car garages, and yes, even our diseases. The line between what the mind can and cannot control has gotten very blurry lately, is my point, and so how can a person confronted with such a pointed rebuke as the one that Elizabeth and I were dealing with—barrenness, for heaven's sake, oldest curse in the book—*not* be haunted by the notion that their failure is some outward manifestation of an inward corruption?

Or let's leave out all religiously loaded terminology—and this is what I said to that counselor: Forget curses and corruption and divine retribution. The fact was, for six years[3] Elizabeth and I had been called upon on an almost monthly basis to put our heads together, get in touch with our feelings, our resources, our instincts, our savvy, and come up with some way to free ourselves from this prison we were in. And yet for six years running every single plan we came up with had been soundly rejected, left us back where we started, only older, poorer, and more confused. So fine, perhaps we weren't being "punished," but we were receiving a fairly severe critique of our methods.

Or to put it in even more contemporary and acceptable vernacular, there was reason to believe that we might be engaged in an act of protracted self-sabotage.

Now, self-sabotage is not a behavior I would normally have associated with myself, but people change, I guess, and it certainly felt like something had gone awry. Like I'd forgotten something

---

3   We didn't actually start seeing the counselor until very near the end of our bum run.

key—how to choose the things that work, or do the things it took to fix them—all that stuff that used to come fairly naturally.

Thankfully, there did remain one area in which the embers of my former confidence still glowed, where I still believed that could slay the dragon, though I'll admit it was with growing concern now, and an unhealthy sense of reliance, that I took up my sword each morning after coffee.

CHAPTER FOUR

THE WORK

I write for a living—novels mostly; occasionally articles, and I do some screenwriting as well, but it's really the books that wake me up in the morning and put me to bed at night. They tend not to have all that much to do with the life I lead or the world I live in. They're usually set in distant times and far-off places about which I knew very little before I began, which means I spend a lot of time doing research and a lot of time ruminating, and that's pretty much how I was spending my days—professionally—during the years in question.

For the most part, I'd always considered myself very lucky in that—to be able, with the turn of a doorknob and the flick of a desk lamp, to transport myself to some faraway place, to find characters and situations that enchanted me and diverted me, where I could still function with some degree of authority and effectiveness. All that was a godsend. I only wished the same for Elizabeth, that she had somewhere or something to supplant the sense of loss that we were both suffering. She had her teaching, of course, and the summer theater camp she runs. No one who watched her for two minutes in either context would question her talent or commitment—those are all very lucky children. Still, I don't think her profession was ever quite as integral to her sense of who she is. Not as much as motherhood, anyway. She once revealed to me that when she was a little girl, she used to scooch over to one side of her bed at night to make room for her imaginary husband and their imaginary child. That's kind of all you need to know. She had been thinking of herself as a mother, literally dreaming of that day, her whole life. To be denied that dream by fate, by biology, by the clock—whatever the cause was—was to be denied the very gift she believed was her destiny, and the fullest expression of her being: to give.

I, on the other hand, born a man and therefore at a slightly farther remove from the ground and rhythm of the universe, had cultivated a sense of identity that was almost entirely bound up with the typically vain attempt to leave my mark in some more artificial way. And I will admit that in our darker, more dire moments, I did take consolation in that, the fact that no matter how important fatherhood was to me, no matter how much I was willing to sacrifice in order to find out what it meant, I had never looked upon it as the ultimate, or even as the defining, measure of my existence. I always operated on the assumption that, aside from the people I've known and the loved ones who'll survive me, it's what happened behind those doors and beneath those lamps— or what I emerge with, I should say—that would be my legacy, and that it would represent the best I could do. That was always the deal.

And yet of course there were respects in which the whole idea of balancing IVF treatment with novel writing may not have been the best-laid plain. We don't need to go into all the shop-talk reasons why, except to say that both writing and IVF are profoundly isolating, low-percentage maneuvers, whose ultimate success or failure isn't really that open to interpretation. At some point I would find out whether my efforts had succeeded—would know Life and survive and therefore be justified—or whether they were bound to wither and waste away in some dark, silent place.

It was something of a challenge, then, trying to keep the overwhelming sense of loss and futility that was subsuming my reproductive efforts from spilling over into my work, especially since a career in fiction writing is an odd thing to assess. In point of fact, I think most people who aspire to do the things I do would have been generally pleased with the station I'd attained, but as I say, a lot depends upon the standards you apply, and the gauges you use—and I was starting to have doubts. Creatively, I felt like I was doing . . . okay. Under the circumstances. Sometimes I felt like I was grinding my gears a little, but it was hard to tell if that was a function of Elizabeth's and my struggles, or just the fact that writing well is hard. If you don't on some level feel that you're failing your material, you should probably go find some new material.

On the more "professional" side of the ledger, however— where things like money, recognition, and "market penetration" get weighed in—I can't say as I was quite so philosophical. I did have bills to pay, after all, habits to feed, and a sense of purpose to maintain, and on that score I have to confess my feelings tended to run more in the area of grave disappointment verging on embarrassment. I reminded myself that Good Seed Keeps, and I never lost faith that my ship would eventually come in, someday. Still, a good dozen years in, and with four or five books under my belt, it seemed to me the whole project was still coughing and sputtering along at a rate that no self-respecting professional would find remotely acceptable. I wasn't satisfied. Often when I glanced over at the shelf in my office, at the six or seven inches set aside for my personal oeuvre, I felt as if I might have been looking at five little corpses lined up in a row, like the infant mummies of Guanajuato, all dressed up in frills and collars, probably quite handsome in their day, and round and rosy and ready to go, but only in another world, apparently—in this one they evidently hadn't made it past the crawling stage.

Or to put it another, perhaps more apt, way, it sometimes felt that no matter where I turned, I was being made to watch gorgeous grade-A fertilized eggs—little pockets of life in which I had literally invested my all—failing to implant, not taking, shriveling and dying, and no one could really tell me why.

———

But what is so curious, and the reason I bring it up (in addition to the fact that I guess there did appear to be a pattern of dysfunction forming—in my mind at least) is that these two staggering disappointments affected me so differently.

The fertility woes, well, they were a shared burden, of course, and maybe that's the whole deal right there, that I didn't feel I was bearing all the blame and therefore felt justified in sidestepping some of the coals. But it also seemed clear to me that what was happening at these doctors' offices and clinics fell squarely into the category of "things I cannot change." Yes, Elizabeth and I could try to marshal the best resources we could, we could pray, make informed decisions, eat pumpkin seeds, stink up our kitchens with putrid tea blends, and perform our little ritual with the needles and swabs every night at six thirty, but for myself, I still recognized that whatever became of these efforts, they were basically cards from a deck. They sucked, but I felt in no position to complain too much, having been dealt flushes and full houses for the first thirty-five years of my life. I didn't resent them. Rarely if ever did they rouse me to anger.

Well, once maybe. I was Rollerblading. This was back when Elizabeth and I were living near Riverside Park, in a one-bedroom apartment which, for all its charms, will (I hope) go down as the saddest place we ever lived; we were sad there so much and so often. I spent a lot of time down by the Hudson River blading my frustration away, and it happened one time that My Lord and Maker, God, on top of everything else he was doing to foil me and my good intentions, had the temerity to blow wind in my face not only on the southbound leg of my route, but then, when I turned around and started skating north again, I could swear that sonofabitch shifted wind and hit me head-on with a downright gale, which, as anyone who Rollerblades knows, kind of takes the fun out.

Well, that was it. That was the last straw. Down there by the river, bundled up in my scarf and ski cap and sweatpants, and with the howling wind as my cover, I hauled off and gave God the what-for, told him he could kiss my ass; eat this, suck that, shove that up there and spin. Basically I told him I thought he was a punk, that I was sick of his bullshit, his deliberately capricious give-and-take, bait-and-switch approach to life and karma, but that he should take no satisfaction in the crap he'd been pulling lately because he hadn't laid a glove on me. I told him he could keep on with these cheap shots all he liked—he clearly didn't know who he was dealing with—whom, excuse me—because I was going to kick his ass anyway. As he was my witness, I was going to show him. Bitch. I think I may have spit a few times.

So I was pretty well exhausted by the time I got back to the 107th Street exit, and cold and drenched, but I think it was good, actually, that we had that talk. I think he respected me a lot more after that.

But that was the only time, I swear, that I went so far as to point a finger, index or otherwise, at God or anyone else regarding the whole fertility fiasco. Even in the face of our more human agents, the doctors at all these clinics, I bore no particularly hard feelings. I could see they were trying. There were times I felt their focus wasn't all it could have been—their services were in such demand—but there was deliberate care and effort being taken, and when things didn't work out, I believe they felt authentic sympathy for us, and we felt for them. We were killing their stats, after all.

———

My attitude toward what was going on over at my publisher was another matter entirely. Maybe because one tends to think of one's career as something one *can* control, something one is *supposed* to control, but whatever the reason, I did not for one second regard the commercial performance of my books to be a card from a deck. I regarded it as a direct consequence of what struck me at the time as being a manifestly anemic, shoe-shuffling, shoulder-shrugging, and frankly horseshit performance on their part—

But let me stop right here and say I know. I know you've heard this one, or if you haven't, God bless you, you must not know any authors, because the fact is, 99 percent of us feel this way 100 percent of the time. It's just the nature of the business, I'm afraid, of competing for attention in a dwindling market, and the fact that the kind of extended focus it takes to write a book winds up giving those who do it for a living all the perspective of a mole-rat. So be assured that even as I sit here, I am keenly aware of that probably apocryphal but no less entertaining story about the time Marsha Mason was overheard in a New York City restaurant screaming at Neil Simon about how he had "ruined" her career!

Thankfully, my purpose here is not to justify or to defend my outrage. It is simply to convey how all this—the most significant ongoing relationship in my professional life (the span of which coincided almost exactly with the time Elizabeth and I had been together, courtship included)—was making me *feel*, how it was *affecting* me, and the answer, I'm afraid to say, was not good. I was very angry, and oftentimes a lot worse than that—like fit-to-be-tied, chop-down-a-forest, pound-a-tunnel-through-that-mountain pissed, just at the sheer ongoing waste of it all.

For the most part I tried to be a fair player and direct most of this anger at my own self—for not having been more aggressive, or taken more personal responsibility for the selling of my wares; they were *my* wares, after all. But I'd be lying if I said there weren't a few others I included in the indictment—colleagues, associates at the house in whom I guess I felt I'd placed too much stock, from whom I heard what I wanted to hear. When not cursing my native lack of salesmanship, it was in their general direction that I did most of my venting, foot-stomping, spitting, and speechifying.

Not in person, mind you, and never out loud. I remained pretty hail-fellow-well-met in their presence, because I knew— these voices in my head were probably just that, my demons talking. For the most part, I tried to be a gentleman, count my blessings, keep my nose to the grindstone, all that. But as the years passed and titles came and went to diminishing returns, those demons definitely got louder. I couldn't quell the sense that this whole arrangement—my professional situation—was essentially rotten, ill-conceived. No progress was being made, nothing substantial was being built. I began to feel used, duped, taken for granted, all those sorts of things one feels when one feels one is being treated shabbily—including discouraged. For the first time in my life I began to wonder if maybe I wasn't as good as I thought I was, and the sad part is that I actually found this idea kind of consoling, that maybe this, this fledgling existence, was as much I could ever have expected, given what I did and how I did it. I vastly preferred that to the notion that I had screwed up my career with bad decisions, or that I'd trusted the wrong people—because that, as I say, just drove me nuts. And yet for the life of me I couldn't figure out what the truth was. I could achieve no lasting perspective, or clarity, or peace of mind. My anger was like an infection that wouldn't go away, or like a charcoal briquette that had somehow been lodged in my brain, and every time I thought it might have finally died, I'd pass a bookstore, or see something in a magazine, and the damn thing would flare up again, and cost me another two man-hours.

And I guess you don't have to be Sigmund Freud. I could see now, those trips to the clinic had made it pretty clear somehow: I was mortal. My time was limited; my product, more finite than I could ever have imagined. These books were how I'd chosen to be of use, and I'd bet the house on them, at the expense of everything else I might have done instead. That's how sure I'd been; I had no back-up. But here I was, thirty-five, thirty-six, thirty-seven years old, and despite my best efforts, what I had to give wasn't proving to be of much use at all. Whoever's fault it was, the gamble was failing right before my eyes, and so the sense of loss, of wasted effort and squandered opportunity just kept eating at me . . . well, I was going to say "every day," but the truth is it ate at me every moment of every day, except for when I was actually at my desk writing, or injecting Elizabeth with her evening dose of Lupron.

CHAPTER FIVE

THE LAST STAND

So we did try donor-egg IVF. That was kind of our last stand in the world of Assisted Reproductive Technology. Donor-egg IVF is where the couple in question pays to have multiple eggs harvested from a third party, the *donor*, so that those presumably healthy eggs can be fertilized with the husband's sperm and then transferred at the appropriate moment back into the womb of the wife.

You might want to read that twice.

Our doctor had actually been alluding to the procedure for a couple of years—you know, worse comes to worst, he said, it was pretty sure-fire—but we basically covered our ears and la-la-la'd whenever he'd brought it up. The whole idea was just too through-the-looking-glass.

But I guess it's tribute to just how elastic our thinking had become after seven failed IVFs, the donor-egg version started to look not so crazy. We toyed with the idea of "unknown" donors. We even looked at a few applications, handwritten forms from young women offering their eggs anonymously. They all sounded very nice and properly motivated ("I have a sister who went

through infertility problems, so I know how hard it can be . . . "),
but when we found ourselves rejecting candidates because we
didn't like their penmanship or because for some reason they
seemed a little "too eager," we did begin wonder if this was the
right thing for us.

We'd probably have put the whole idea to rest had there not
emerged from within Elizabeth's side of the family a potential
"known" donor. And I don't want to say too much about her for
the sake of her privacy, except that we obviously wouldn't have
proceeded if we hadn't had complete faith in her. From the
moment Elizabeth called her and broached the subject, gently,
her response was incredibly attuned, cautious but open. To the
extent one can have an instinct about such a thing, she showed a
remarkable one. She understood what it was we had been going
through, the extents and the limits of the role we were asking her
to play. We all agreed that the best way to think about this was as
a gift—a donation, like the name said—something she had it in
her power to give that we needed in order to be a family. Maybe.
How the gesture would unfold from there, how the genetic element would play out in years to come, and manifest itself—in hair
color, in gesture, a particular way of laughing—there was no way
of knowing obviously, and no way of knowing how we would all
react, cope with the possible conflicts and jealousies. We just had
to trust. Her. And each other. And the child. And honesty.

We didn't get our hopes up, or bring any undue expectation to
the process. By that point, we were beyond trying to design the
future. We were just looking for what worked. So we took the
leap, pretty blind, but not alone this time. And the trust we placed
in her, our kin, was more than vindicated, as over the course of

the next three or four months, she underwent all the same shots and bruises and bandages that Elizabeth had. She had to flip her schedule and come to New York, stay in what wasn't much better than a flea-bag hotel because that's all we could afford at the time, take all those sonograms and painful, invasive procedures, all for us and without a murmur of complaint. Really, she proved to be every bit as gracious, selfless, faith restoring, and evidently fertile as we could ever have hoped, which only made the outcome that much more depressing. It would have been nice to keep those genes in the family, but no. No dice. Even after all that, giving up on Elizabeth's genetic legacy, assuming the risk and all the unintended emotional consequences that might follow, trusting love to see us and our would-be family through, even after that, the Fates looked down and shook their heads again.

PART TWO

ADOPTION

CHAPTER SIX

ADOPTION, IN PROSPECT

So that is what brought us to the threshold of adoption: Not inspiration. Not conviction. But an incredibly painful and exhausting process of elimination.

Of course, we had been looking into it, on and off, just to get the lay of the land. We had toured some websites, attended some introductory meetings, and all the experts seemed to agree that we should probably get the biological aspirations out of our system before proceeding. They said adoption was far too sacred and demanding an undertaking to be entered into as a mere contingency, and that's definitely true, but it also points to what is one of the more unfortunate unintended consequences of reproductive technology: that by extending indefinitely a couple's hopes of having their own biological child, RT casts adoption in the role of Perennial Plan B. It becomes that thing you'll do, that bridge you'll cross, if this doesn't work out. So making the transition, trying to drum up the same energy, the same excitement, the same hope you'd been bringing to *in vitro* for all those years requires real mental gymnastics.

A couple years into the process, at a point in time when Elizabeth and I were already fully committed and expecting a child, I was out in California visiting an old friend, Tim. I had gone to meet him and his distractingly good-looking six-year-old son out along the park paths that border the beach at Santa Monica, and we'd been discussing what Elizabeth and I were waiting on, the various hows and wherefores of adopting internationally. Tim was being characteristically open and generous. Looking out at the ocean, he began shaking his head at one point—admiringly. He said he had a lot of friends who were going through "the whole infertility thing," and he just wished for their sake that they could move on and open up to what we were doing.

There was an awkward silence. I appreciated the sentiment, of course, but it made me a little uncomfortable, which he must have sensed. A week or so later he sent me an e-mail apologizing if he had misspoken; he realized it was a sensitive topic and all. I wrote back and told him not to worry about it, but that he probably shouldn't be giving us too much credit, since we'd traveled a pretty long road getting to where we were. What I didn't say is that we were still on the road, and it still felt awfully steep to me.

And that is not the only time I've heard biological parents wonder at the seeming reluctance of their less fertile friends to adopt. Not too long after that, I was out at a restaurant—a birthday party with arranged seating—and one of my table mates was expressing the same idea, but even more directly and earnestly: What is it, she asked, with what seemed to be complete sincerity, that kept them—us, she meant, the reproductively challenged—from embracing adoption sooner? I'm not sure I would have answered—her husband sidled over and interrupted the conversation (something about the babysitter)—but if I had replied, I suspect it would have been something along the lines of, "Well, because adopting a child is clearly the most difficult and horrifying thing that two people can do together."

It is. I firmly believe that. In fact, part of the reason I'd deep down known all along that it was going to come to this was because I'd already identified adoption as being just about the hardest thing I could imagine (and therefore my destiny). And not just because giving up on one's own genetic legacy is hard, or that giving yourself over to another completely unknown genetic legacy is a little terrifying. Even setting that stuff aside, I could see that the actual nuts-and-bolts process of adopting was intensely daunting; much more than IVF.

It was just as expensive, don't kid yourself. It was apparently way more tedious. It usually took longer, sometimes *much* longer, and there was no guarantee it would work, in the short term or the long. A brief tour of the Internet will show: tales of adoption woe are as endless as they are varied, but the reasons all boil down to the same simple truth: prospective adoptive parents are desperate, they have very little legal recourse, and no leverage.

In other words, people can act all they want like everyone loves adoption so why don't more of us do it; the fact is we remain a society—we are a *species*, let's face it—that prizes the blood-bond *über Alles*. And the law makes that pretty clear. In the courtroom, biology trumps deed and good intentions almost every time. Even distant grandparents can wedge a child from the arms of adopted parents just by showing up in court. And biological mothers, forget about it. Why, did you know that in certain states, a pregnant woman can enter into a contractual agreement with a prospective adoptive couple whereby the couple pays all that woman's expenses, medical bills, and late-night Whopper runs; compensates her for hours lost from her job and basically foots the bill for everything she needs through the healthy delivery of the child, at which point the biological mother can change her mind, keep the baby, and not have to pay back the prospective couple one red cent?

Call me paranoid, but that didn't strike me as being a very inviting legal climate.

Moreover—and again, this is all on the *domestic* front—it seemed like the post-delivery agreements being drawn up between adoptive and biological parents were leaning heavily in favor of what's called "open" adoption, where the biological mother is granted a level of ongoing access to her offspring—through update letters, report cards, scheduled visits, etc.—that, taken to certain extremes, made the whole thing seem like one giant free-babysitting scam. That's not to cast aspersions. I have no doubt that the vast majority of birth mothers are noble young women making the most difficult decision of their lives, and I respect the fact that they were doing so for the sake of their children. That *is* the ultimate sacrifice. And I am equally sure that there are many couples out there for whom the idea of open adoption, even wide open adoption, is no problem—and who knows whether it's better or worse for the children; everyone is different. But for us, the issue was fairly clear-cut. Just because we'd been through the IVF wars and lost, that didn't mean that Elizabeth should always have to save an extra seat at the dance recital.

―――――

Alas, over in the realm of international adoption, our early research revealed a landscape just as forbidding. There, the prerogative of the biological mother to change her mind with impunity had been replaced by the prerogative of a state bureaucracy to change its mind with impunity, which happens a lot—and I mean *a lot*—as said bureaucracy tries to maintain some balance between the needs of the children, the capacity of its orphanages, and the pressure of virulent local interest groups, who regard it as a shameful blight upon their nation's reputation that their most precious natural resource is being flown out of the country every day in the grateful arms of well-off Americans. Boo-hiss. That, as well as good old-fashioned corruption (because there is money in the sale of children, after all), makes foreign adoption a highly politically charged, harrowing, and uncertain bet, which finds thousands of innocent couples losing years of their lives waiting on children they may never bring home.

So there was that.

―――――

Moving from the legal arena to the cultural—from the classroom to the playground, if you will—the situation didn't get a whole lot better. Finding out that you were adopted is a punchline proxy for the worst thing that can happen to a kid. Telling your brother he was adopted is a way of being mean. At the time we started our paperwork, packaged stories about children being reunited with their "real" parents was becoming a kind of cottage industry, cheap heartwarming entertainment churned out for the fat fertile masses, all while the adoptive—or as I would strongly suggest they be called, "actual"—parents of all these children-now-made-whole were left to gaze on silently through rainy windowpanes, alone.

Am I being melodramatic? A little defensive? You bet I am, but that's my point. Adoptive parents and their children *are* intensely sensitive creatures whose feelings simply aren't shown a lot of respect, as much as we pretend otherwise.

I was on the subway one time, and this must have been when Elizabeth and I were just dipping our toes. A bunch of teenagers got on, college freshmen, clearly all just getting to know one another. One revealed that she was adopted. Actually, her roommate yielded up the information—"Yeah, she was adopted." My ears perked up. The young woman in question gave it a kind of "big whoop" shrug—yeah, it's true—to which one of the boys replied, *first thing out of his mouth*, "Oh yeah? So have you tried to contact your real parents?" I damn near took him out at his knees. I should have, on behalf of the girl's actual parents, but I doubt anyone in the car would have had the slightest idea what I was doing. He was just trying to get in her pants, after all; show some interest.

Still, that was a first for me, feeling the sting of mere words, but there's no denying: Depending upon the ears that hear it, that phrase "real parents" is right up there with "nigger" and "cunt." Except that no one out there seems to be remotely aware.

And mind you, those are just the hurdles we encountered *out there*. There was also the baggage we were bringing—opinions and prejudices we barely knew we had, but now were forced to consider in earnest.

The whole Nature vs. Nurture issue: Are our identities more or less biologically determined, or are we molded by circumstance? And what is the dynamic between the two? In the past, my position had always been that this was a classically bogus distinction: that insofar as neither Nature nor Nurture had ever managed to exert one photon's worth of influence on the world—that is, on the given moment—without the complete and utter consent of the other, the two were for all intents and purposes indistinguishable, so why bother with such metaphysical nonsense (other, I guess, than to make public policy)?

Well, I was right, of course, don't get me wrong. Still, when you find yourself considering adoption in earnest, you are forced to admit the common-sense meaning of the distinction, and in my case, I had to admit that in my heart of hearts I'd always been something of a naturist. (By nature, a naturist; though raised to be a nurturist.) My experience taught me that most people are who they are without regard to what's going on around them— that we all possess inborn resonant frequencies, if you will, that act as divining rods in guiding us along, and will eventually lead us to compatible or harmonious frequencies in one way or another. To put it another way, you could wake up tomorrow to a nuclear winter or as heir to the Palace at Versailles, I say it would take you about three hours before you begin experiencing all the same basic levels of irritation, comfort, ambition, and sloth as you always did, because those are the levels that make you feel at home.

What did that have to do with adoption? Just that when I looked at a baby, I didn't see lovable *tabula rasa*. I saw Distinct Other, and I figured the chances of my getting along with that baby were about the same as my chances of getting along with any stranger on the street. Maybe that makes me a terrible person, or maybe there's nothing so radical in that opinion, but it does go to show what a hair-raising crapshoot I considered adoption to be: Take how you felt meeting your freshman year roommate for the first time, and raise the stakes by about forty billion.

So that was the bad news, I guess.

The good news is that adoption was not strange to me. I have two cousins who were adopted, sisters, about my age, and from them I took two important lessons—little did I know when I was learning them:

First is that when it comes to family, I guess I really *don't* think it matters so much whether you share a blood connection, since the cousins I'm thinking of were the cousins I was closest to growing up. We all lived in New York, saw each other at all appropriate holidays, sledded together, swam together, played house, and Monopoly and Doctor together. If you asked me who my cousins were, they're the ones I'd have thought of first, and never did it occur to me that they were less related to me than say, my blood cousins who lived in Arizona whom I saw maybe once every three years. The only difference was that we couldn't get into all those conversations about who got whose nose, or sneeze, or ugly feet, but that was okay. Along with sunsets and mortgage rates, children, in their infinite wisdom, don't really care about such things.

The second lesson goes somewhat hand in hand with what I was saying about Nature up there, and the fact that I think we are who we are come hell or high water, and that is my sense that a given child's experience of adoption—that is, of being someone who was adopted—is an almost entirely individual matter. I don't really think anything meaningful can be said, categorically, about adopted children. It's like talking about "Israeli public opinion." There are six million of them. And one of the reasons I'm fairly sure of that—in addition to the fact that I've tuned my ears to the topic the last several years—is because I know, for instance, that the younger of the two cousins, when she was around twenty or so, decided to seek out her biological mother. I don't believe she ended up finding her, but I completely understand the impulse, and don't see that it diminishes the service, the love, or the claim of her actual parents, my uncle and my aunt.[1]

Anyway, the older of these two sisters did *not* seek out her biological mother. On the contrary, she was *sought out* by her biological mother. The woman found her and wanted to get in touch. My cousin told her, no, I already know my parents; basically she hung up the phone. And I can understand that too. I don't think either her choice or her sister's choice was better or worse, just very different, and having known them both their whole lives,

---

1   My two aunts, in fact: my cousins were adopted by my uncle and his first wife, my mother's sister, who passed away in 1974. My uncle remarried to a woman who entered the fold with seamless individual grace, which goes to show that not only is "cousin" a matter of heart not blood, so is "aunt."

their choices strike me as being perfectly in keeping with who they are, and that's what I'm getting at. Same roof, same rules, same food, they still managed to find themselves all along the way, very different people who obviously entertain radically different attitudes toward their biological roots. And any time I've spoken to other adopted children, I'm impressed by the same moral: there is no moral. There is no norm.

And that is good news, I think.

CHAPTER SEVEN

GETTING STARTED

So, for reasons I've already touched upon, Elizabeth and I had decided to go with international, rather than domestic, adoption. The first meeting we ever attended was at a highly respected agency located in an Upper East Side brownstone, just a very general, so-you-think-you-wanna-adopt-type thing, with cookie trays and coffee tanks and testimonials. But that was where we got our first real taste of what international adoption is really all about—at the outset, at least—and that is making choices.

Granted, there had been a lot of choosing involved with IVF—which method, which month, which drug—but at least there had been doctors around to advise us, experts with certificates on the wall. And once the choices were made, we got to act on them and see results; there were the syringes and sonograms. Here, we were just presented with a laundry list of variables we had to consider—features of our potential child's background that would help guide us in our thinking—and handed a pencil and a pad. It was a little like Off Track Betting.

The variables were clear at least. They were:

> race
>
> nationality
>
> length of wait
>
> expense
>
> age
>
> gender
>
> medical risk

A bunch of factors that, if all goes well and love prevails, will end up having very little to do with the relationship you forge with your child, he or she being an individual first, not a gender, race, expense, or some unforeseen medical condition waiting to unfold. And yet a decision must be made. You literally cannot move forward without answering these questions and putting them in order, and you can't do that without feeling terribly cheap, impatient, selfish, cowardly, or bigoted.

Which is to say nothing of the fact that, after four years of having every tack we tried denied, denied, and denied again, my faith in Elizabeth's and my judgment was at a pretty low ebb. I wouldn't have put us in charge of ordering a pizza.

Just to give you an example; Remember that apartment hunt right before the miscarriage? Well, we still had to find a place. Maybe three weeks after the D&C we were back on the streets, chasing down For Rent ads in the paper, and we came upon an okay railroader down on Second Avenue. Small, but with an extra room for me to work in, and one for the baby, should wonders never cease. We were getting a little panicked about finding a place, and the landlady seemed very nice. She owned a jewelry store right around the corner, so we told her yes, we'll take it. We heaved a big mutual sigh of relief, then went off to get some lunch and the security deposit.

In the diner, Elizabeth started talking about the apartment, and all of a sudden it sounded like she hadn't liked it all that much. I said, Didn't you? She admitted, not really, she'd only gone with it because she thought I liked it. I told her the only reason I'd gone with it was because it seemed like *she* liked it. I got a little ticked, as I think in this instance she really had been misleading in the apartment, but that is neither here nor there. Faced with the prospect of moving somewhere that neither of us actually wanted to live, we solved the problem like any self-respecting couple would, by retro-fudging the numbers on our financial statement to make us look so broke and so in debt that the owner's management agency would reject the agreement. Which they did, thank God. Sometimes it pays to be poor.

So anyway, yes, choosing a child. Or at least, choosing our priorities. For us, after all we'd been through, the most important thing was clearly health. Elizabeth had worked in an orphanage in Tijuana when she was in college. She also had a student when she first started teaching in San Francisco, a boy with leukemia whom she tutored in-home for about a year. She'd grown close to him. She watched him die. That, plus the four years we'd just gone through in and out of hospitals and clinics, definitely inclined us to want to play it safe when it came to health. Priority #2? Probably age—the younger the better. #3? Speed. Enough with the waiting. Looking back, our priorities make it pretty clear, we were two people sick and tired of this chapter of their life, and desperately wanting to turn the page.

And that page, the new page—given our abiding concerns—was filled with Asian faces: Korean, Cambodian, Chinese. The agency folk didn't say it in so many words, but Eastern Europe and Russia definitely came off as high-risk. The waits could be extended. The children tended to be older and not as healthy. Medical histories were scant. There was a lot of drinking and smoking in that part of the world. The orphanages were over-burdened. The paperwork was mountainous. The money, esti-mable, and that wasn't even counting what happened under the table.

A place like Korea, on the other hand, sounded like just what the doctor ordered. Clean. Fast. Reliable medical backgrounds. Young children, six months. Heck, they said you didn't even have to go there if you didn't want to. Not that we would have consid-ered such a thing—that just seems impolite. Still, the idea of the doorbell ringing and being handed a healthy child had its appeal.

So it seemed like that's where we were probably leaning. Dur-ing the show-and-tell portion of that first meeting, a recent adop-tive mother brought out her son, of Korean descent. He appeared to be somewhere between six months and ten thousand years old. Dear God, he was cute, and wise and alert and Buddhaesque. He looked at us and smiled. Elizabeth nudged me, and I was right with her. We'd have snatched him there and made a run for it if she hadn't been wearing heels.

But one other thing happened in that first meeting that would stick in my craw long after. At one point during the question-and-answer session, one of the other prospective mothers had raised her hand and made reference to the children who'd been adopted through the agency as being "lucky." I wouldn't have thought twice about it, but it made sense: life in a Guatemalan orphanage versus life on the Upper East Side of Manhattan—I think we could all see what she was getting at. But it was as if someone had said "Macbeth" in a theater. The agency representatives all went stiff-lipped and quiet. Then one of them actually spoke up and said they discouraged our thinking of the children as "lucky."

Again, I supposed I could see her point. You don't want to found a relationship on the idea that someone is doing someone else a favor. But it did strike me, almost the scolding nature of the correction, and to this day I'm not 100 percent sure I understand. Luck is not a zero-sum game, after all. Couldn't we *all* think of ourselves as lucky?

But I think the real reason it stuck with me is because that may have been the first time it occurred to me that we were no longer the aggrieved party here. For four years, it seemed like we'd been the sick ones, the ones in need. Now I realized there were the children, too, and it's not that that was such a revelation. Perhaps it simply goes to show what a peculiar place the IVF-scarred couple is coming from. Or maybe I should just speak for myself, but I was not there at that meeting because this was something I had always thought about doing; I was not there because my biological spawn were all grown and I wanted to fill the void; I was not there because I'd been inspired by an ad on TV or an article about Angelina Jolie; I was not there, that is to say, for the sake of the children. I was there for exactly the same reason I'd been going to those clinics for the last four years: because I was hoping that maybe this would be what worked, because I refused to let some accident of fate, some mysterious biological glitch, keep Elizabeth and me from what we still regarded as our con-joined destiny, and our hope—to be parents.

And again, there's nothing that says such thinking excludes the idea of helping children in need, but it does introduce a certain dissonance to the proceedings, and I could hear it that first meeting—like two voices vying for my attention, laying bare the conflict that lies right at the heart of adoption, and that would continue to stir and trouble my conscience for several years to come.

There was the one that said the point of all of this, the beating we'd been taking, had clearly been for us to get over ourselves, strip us of all false notions of what we thought we wanted or what would be good for us. Life, in its eternal wisdom, had brought us to a very humble place of withoutness, leaving us no real choice but the happiest, which was to commit ourselves completely and utterly to whatever was given us; to force us to recognize that *all* that matters is the care and attention we bring to the individual and to the moment, and the only thing we can do in preparation for that moment is to open our hearts and purify them, burn them free of all bias and expectation. Trust in love, be its medium, and proceed.

The alternative view, of course, is that that is complete bullshit. We had come to a place where nature and spontaneity had left us high and dry. This was *not* the time to abandon our discriminative abilities or our instincts. They were all that we had left—the capacity to figure out what we wanted and how we were going to get it, and fuck anyone who tried to move us from our path. They've got their own agenda, which nine times out of ten is getting the number of my bank account. Decisions had to be made here. We could not let that New Age hokum, other people's politics or notions of right and wrong, or liberal guilt affect our thinking one whit. There were no right or wrong ways to think about any of this. There was only how honest we were willing to be with ourselves. If we want something, we should go get it. If we're uncomfortable with something, we should recognize it, change it, react to it, because if we don't, and we go ahead and do something for someone *else's* good reason, we are going to pay for it for the rest of our lives, and so is the child. Do not judge yourself. Know yourself, and proceed accordingly.

Those were the poles of the axis around which my brain would spin for the next couple of years; those, the two advisors on my shoulders: Jesus and Alec Baldwin, and it was with their voices in my head that I now contemplated the various factors that had been laid out before us, from which we would be cobbling together our course.

So, Korea, then? China? Did I not, on some level, want a girl? Weren't girls less scary than boys? Or is that the stupidest thing anyone ever thought? Does it matter, my former relationship with people of similar descent? Should it matter, my innate interest in the history and the culture of the place? And if we decided we did want to take on the various challenges of being a family of manifestly mixed race, did that mean we should plan on remaining in big metropolitan areas where there are lots of interracial families? Does that matter? Do any of these questions matter, or are they just the stuff you're left to think about until such time as the child arrives, at which point you'll be so knee-deep in diapers, and so swept away by the actual individual person in front of you that all such concerns will drift away like the abstract nonsense they ultimately are? I tended to think yes, but until that child arrived, one way or the other, the abstract nonsense was all I had.

And not all the nonsense was so abstract. When I went out on my lunch runs now, I found myself stepping out into a whole new world. This city, my home, this heretofore blessed sea of strangers, had suddenly transformed into a world populated by potential sons and or daughters—or people who might bear a striking resemblance to them, at any rate. My daily walk to the sandwich shop had become a stroll through the kingdom of potential heirs. Might my boy have that nose there? That unbecoming snarl? Be six foot three? Have those bowed legs? Who knows? That cluster at the corner, waiting for the light—the Guatemalan teenager headed to the park with a soccer ball.

"Son! Let me carry that for you. How was the flight?"

The Chinese girl, a student—so quiet and demure.

"Did you get the paper done on time? Of course you did. I'm proud of you."

The restless Filipino on the delivery bike. The Ukrainian driving that cab.

Did I have it in me to be the father of every single one of these people, to be equally calm and open and patient, to be as fierce in my love as a parent should be? You never know until you try, I guess, and I did my best to keep an open mind, but I'll be honest with you, those couple of blocks never did wonders for my appetite.

———

I'm not sure I made the connection in my head—I'm not sure there was a connection to be made—but it would have been around this time that my latest book came out, the one that had been conceived and written entirely in the context of our reproductive trials.

I wasn't getting my hopes up. In going over the galleys, I'd already come to recognize that this book represented a fairly writerly performance, so I had prepared myself for another round of the house's flattest champagne. Or I thought I had, but I guess not. If a book's release might be compared to an object falling toward the surface of lake, my fifth zipped down through like polished stone. When I say no splash, I'm not kidding. Outside of reviews, which were actually pretty good, there was nothing—not a reading, not a radio spot, not a mention in a magazine. Zip. And I am here to tell you, no matter how accustomed one becomes to the writer's rhythm of endless toil and fleeting thanks, it remains the case that to put that amount of work into something—four years, in this instance, locked away in a room, researching, composing, sanding, polishing, bringing everything to standard—and upon successful completion of the mission, to be denied even a single opportunity to speak on its behalf—this is, in a word, damaging.

And I knew it meant my relationship with the house was over—by mutual consent, I'm sure, but from my end I knew, books are too hard. To get them done, you have to believe that what you're doing matters, and I simply could not have sustained that belief through the completion of another manuscript, not knowing that when I was done I'd be handing it to the same people again.

Too bad, too. Because I was actually at this time also homing in on what my next big project was going to be. Two or three ideas had been competing for my attention, but a clear leader was now emerging. As usual, the one that seemed impossible. I could tell already, this one made everything I'd done up to that point look like chopsticks. To get it done, I knew I would need to work with people I could trust, and who respected me and believed in what I was doing. In other words, I knew that for the time being at least, I would be working alone.

———

Anyway, back to the story. One day, I was out skating in the park and I had a semi-lucid moment. I was cutting from east to west at around 80th Street, headed for the Great Lawn, when I happened by the statue of Jagiello, King of Lithuania, Duke of Poland. It's a big one, life-size. He's mounted on an armored horse, wearing a fish-scale breastplate; holding two enormous swords high above his head, crossed. Feature for feature, he looks a little like the Statue of Liberty's brother, and definitely the one who got the better of the bargain.

And I don't know that I can say it was one of those signs I was talking about—when you're as familiar with Central Park as I am, "chancing" by a statue is a fairly voluntary act—but I did feel a definite tug as I passed by. I actually whirled around him a couple times, and just seeing the words on his pedestal, the large chiseled "Lithuania" on one side, "Poland" on the other, I felt a stirring in me, I did. Call it the call of the cold-earth peoples. I realized that maybe for some it didn't matter so much where their child came from. To me it did. Who was I kidding? I spend most of my days and nights trolling underground rivers and streams, currents taking me all kinds of places, places that fascinate me and enchant me and haunt me and invade me, and it was important to me that my child's homeland be one of those places. As I gazed up at Jagiello's dark scowl, there was no question in my mind that I could find my way somewhere beneath the Carpathian mountains. Easy.

That day, when Elizabeth got home from work, we spoke. I told her what I'd been thinking, that it still seemed to me that we were going about this wrong; either we could do this by avoiding what we *didn't* want, or we could figure out what we *did* want and go get it. I felt like all our reasons for considering Korea were borne of fear, not excitement—and what excited me was the idea of adopting a child from a part of the world to which I felt a visceral connection. I knew it meant the process was going to be harder, that it was going to entail more risk, more work, and more money, but it just seemed to me that whatever we decided to do, we should do it because it seemed like an adventure; not because it felt safe.

I guess she must have been feeling something similar, because she didn't put up much of an argument. She actually looked a little relieved. The only concern was the process, because Eastern Europe was by all accounts a tougher row to hoe. We'd have to be smarter, she said. More hands-on.

I said, exactly.

CHAPTER EIGHT

ROMANIA?

I am actually, believe it or not, legally proscribed from going into too much detail about what happened over the course of the next year or so, which suits me just fine. Of all the chapters of my life, this is probably the one I'd leave on the cutting room floor, but briefly, and just to connect the dots:

We decided to secure the services of a private adoption lawyer rather than an agency, in the hope that this would grease the wheels a little, maybe give us an inside track. The one we found had done good work in Lithuania—we had a friend who had used her, with smashing success—but when we went out to meet her, she said she'd lost her contact there and the laws had changed. Lithuania had slowed down, but she claimed she'd been having great success in Romania the last few months—very young children, very quick turnaround—and might we be interested in that?

We'd never really thought about Romania, and she must have sensed our hesitation (or noticed the color of my hair). She said if we were at all worried about gypsies, we shouldn't be. I'd never really thought about gypsies either, though her assurance did confirm my sense that the gypsy really is the last bastion of unapologetic prejudice. I asked her how she could be so sure; it didn't seem to me that any country would allow a couple to make that kind of distinction up front. She, who was herself of Eastern European extraction, said she could eyeball it. She walked us over to the corkboard on her office wall. It was covered with photos of children whose adoptions she'd recently facilitated, maybe twenty. She started pointing from face to face.

"Gypsy . . . gypsy . . . no gypsy . . . gypsy . . . no gypsy . . . "

When I recounted this scene to my mother the following day, she asked, "What's wrong with gypsies?"

I said I wasn't sure—maybe having to pack all those crystal balls in your luggage. That, and you probably don't want your own kid trying to pick your pocket all the time.

My mother pointed out that any child trying to pick my pocket was in for a world of disappointment.

I agreed. No gypsy.

But Romania, yes. Why not? It wasn't exactly what we'd been aiming for, but it was close, and let's not forget: Early in our courtship, back when I used to visit Elizabeth in San Francisco, she had very considerately borrowed a friend's little electronic keyboard for me, to make up for the Steinway upright I (entirely serendipitously) was living with in New York at the time. In comparison to the Steinway, the Casio was a little like playing a touch-tone phone, but I decided to make use of it anyway (because this is procrastination we're talking about) by teaching myself some simple pieces I'd always liked. I went to the public library and illegally copied sheet music, smuggled it back to

Elizabeth's apartment, and pecked my way through; I'm not really all that well trained. But the first piece I ever taught myself to play? Only Bartók's first Romanian folk dance, the "Stick Dance."

So, 'nuff said.

But again, I'm not sure how much more I'm allowed to say about what followed, except that what you've heard is somewhat true, and that the process of adopting from a foreign country is a little like playing poker for the first time with your drunk older cousins. The rules keep changing. You're never sure who to trust, and there's a good chance the whole thing will end in tears or scandal.

Basically, Elizabeth and I waited and waited, and waited some more. We'd paid most of the money up front, but didn't actually do much paperwork after that, which probably should have been a clue that something was up. Mostly we made phone calls trying to figure out what was going on, which we never quite did. There were a lot of news reports about corruption and a possible moratorium that might be shutting down Romanian adoption altogether, but our lawyer did a good job of reassuring us with talk of pending legislation and special "exception" lists. How much of it had any basis in fact, I'll never know. Let's just say it was not one of the prouder moments in the history of my healthy skepticism.

But we were trying with all our might to be hopeful. We moved to an apartment near the park with an extra bedroom. I set up a crib. Elizabeth sewed matching curtains and bumpers and pillows; bought baby clothes, girls' clothes, since girls were in the offing. I bought some Dinu Lipatti records. Some Angela Gheorghiu. And every Saturday afternoon at four thirty Elizabeth and I snuggled up on the living room couch together to watch the

Romanian news program on Channel 25. We didn't understand a word, but that wasn't the point. We just wanted to get a look at the people, and try to convince ourselves that this might finally be the answer. This might be what works for us.

Nope. After a year of nothing really making much sense, we started peeking around behind our attorney's back, combing the Internet, and talking to people at the embassies. What we learned was completely disheartening. Basically, the moratorium was for real. No children were getting out of Romania. No exceptions, and our names had never been on any list. The whole thing had been a complete waste of time. And I can see how people of slightly different pathologies than ours might have made a bigger stink, or hung in there, started writing their congressmen, or maybe tried to take on the pretty virulent and xenophobic anti-international adoption lobby that exists in Romania, whose position seems to be that we foreigners want to use their children as sex toys, why else would we spend that kind of money? But it just wasn't a fight we were up for.

We wrote to our attorney to inform her that we were terminating the contract. Not an easy letter to write, that: To the running total of months we'd spent in unstinting pursuit of parenthood without advancing a *single* step in its direction (fifty-two, by my calculation), add another fourteen. It was starting to look like we were just as inept at adopting as we were at conceiving.

We started seeing that counselor—not really a delver, more of a relationship coach—which helped some. I was like a kid at bathtime. I resisted going, I kicked and yelled, but once we got there, I wouldn't stop talking. And maybe I don't really get therapy, but I think it ended in a draw. After ten visits the counselor determined that Elizabeth was sad; I was angry. We both had every reason.

But we still functioned. We ate. We slept. To the big black eye of a space alien documentarian, our behavior was indistinguishable from that of any other culturally programmed automaton. We went to all the movies we were supposed to, bought clothes at the Gap. I traded in my Rollerblades for some jogging sneakers. I started running a lot. A lot. I got back down to the weight I was my senior year of high school, when the trainer for the soccer team pulled me aside and asked if I was feeling all right. Maybe I was, maybe I wasn't. I think I knew at the time, this was just one of those phases that taints everything it touches—the parks, the corners, the sandwich shop. They're all fated to become reminders of how sad you were back then, so tread lightly.

———

But something I found myself thinking about a lot during this period, if you'll pardon a moment of corn, were the touch football games that Nick (then Nicky), Tim (then Timmy), and their father Peter (then Peter) and I used to play in the park. Other people could join in as well and often did—kids, relatives, cousins, uncles, whoever, but the cornerstone rivalry of the games almost always found Timmy and me on one team, and Nicky and Peter on the other. I think it's fair to say that the competitive advantage tilted in favor of Timmy and me, for reasons having mostly to do with growth rates, but also because of one play that Timmy and I had in our arsenal called "The Bomb." The Bomb was no great secret. It was basically a well-synchronized Hail

Mary. Timmy was always quarterback. I was always the receiver. And maybe this is retrospect-painting with a dewy brush—believe me, there are no stats from my life I'd rather see—but it seems to me that The Bomb, conceived as the reception of least likelihood, connected an almost magically high percentage of the time, particularly considering the high-pressure situations for which we assiduously reserved it: A fourth down, field to go, next touchdown wins sort of thing. Tim would only have to look at me in the huddle and give the nod, maybe mouth the word, that's all we needed. We'd break, and I'd mosey up to the line of scrimmage with a deliberately ho-hum air.

And it's still a pretty fresh sense-memory, of Timmy calling hike, Nicky starting the count to three Miss-ippi; Peter backpedaling, already sensing trouble. A couple strides from the line, I'd stutter step, maybe try to sell a quick buttonhook, then roll right and bolt for the end zone as fast as my eleven-year-old legs could carry me. Round about "two Miss-ippi" I'd look back and make eye contact with Timmy just to let him know, "My man is dust; let her rip." At "three Miss-ippi," Nicky would charge over the scrimmage line, arms outstretched and flailing. Timmy might buy an extra second with a quick side-step, then launch the ball— the "Duke," it was called; the name was branded right into the pigskin, quotation marks and all. Timmy would launch the "Duke" just over his younger brother's desperately splayed fingertips.

And I'll say this for Timmy: If there were tighter spirals sailing over the green pastures and frozen tundra of this great land, none was ever more true or elegant. With the majesty of a zeppelin and the fierce purpose of a spear, the "Duke" would head out on its appointed arc, and the sequence of thoughts that would rush through my mind as I raced to track it down are as clear to me now as if we just played this morning.

Thinking first, *No problem, I'll get there, and nothing's in my way.* Looking back again, still confident, but then—

Whoa, maybe not. There was always that moment, too, on a really good Bomb. Maybe just as the "Duke" was reaching its zenith, I'd look up and think, *Wow. Timmy really seems to have put a charge in this one. I don't know if I can—it's definitely going to take one helluva—*

but wait, maybe. . . .

maybe . . .

oh, baby, yes. Extend. Soft hands. Come to Papa.

Tuck. Three more strides, end zone. Game over. *Had it all the way.*

Timmy would call out from the far end of the field, "Yesss!" with arms raised in triumph, while Nicky and Peter hung their heads in dusty despair. A noble effort, once again, but you cannot beat the magic of the Bomb.[2]

---

2   Okay, so it probably isn't fair to glorify such moments without also mentioning one time the Bomb didn't actually connect. I'd managed to outleg my coverage—Peter's brother, John—and it's still possible I might have made the catch had I not collided face-first with the trunk of the tree that was the left corner marker of the end zone, so hard and flush it dislodged the post-operative scab that had formed in the far reaches of my palate, this following the adenoidectomy surgery I'd undergone the day before. After spilling a fair amount of blood there at the roots, I was escorted from the field on wobbly legs and taken to the couch of the Davis apartment, where I was picked up a short while later by my then-trainer, Whitney Hansen. I would not attend the birthday party I had so been looking forward to that evening, but rather spend the rest of the day and night on the living room couch, napping under observation and intermittently vomiting all the blood that had settled and blackened in my stomach. But hey, you gotta pay to play.

But now the reason I found myself thinking about this particular sequence during Elizabeth's and my most dire stretch wasn't for the bygone thrill or the sense of victory, or at least it wasn't *only* that. It was the middle part, that momentary flash of doubt, of thinking maybe I wasn't going to get there this time. I think I just wanted to remind myself that that was okay. A little doubt is fine, good and natural even, *as long as you keep your legs moving.* That was the lesson: those strides you take when you honestly don't think you're going to make it, they're the ones that get you there, and I have Tim to thank for that little insight. Truly, one of my great good fortunes growing up was having a friend who really knew how to lead his receiver. And whose father played an excellent patsy.

═══════

So, boy, did we keep our legs moving. There is an old Russian aphorism: "The cannon shoots far because it does not scatter its shot." Well, around the spring of 2004, Elizabeth and I began attacking our problem with a popcorn machine.

Now that our insurance was finally kicking in on most infertility treatment, we decided to take another crack at that—not IVF, nothing that major, just some intra-uterine injection–type stuff.

Elizabeth had tracked down an adoption agency that claimed to be having some success in Russia. The waits weren't as long and the children weren't as old as we'd been led to expect, so we started paperwork there.

We also made moves toward domestic adoption. As I say, the agencies we'd contacted all tended to encourage a level of openness—to the birth mother—that we weren't comfortable with. We wanted a little more control over whatever contract we drew up with the birth mother, so we secured the services of an*other* lawyer (because, after all, you can't have too many lawyers in your life) and he started advising us on how to go about placing ads in upstate weeklies, twenty words tops: "Child wanted for happy home. . . ." I have to say, that of all the tasks Elizabeth and I were called upon to perform—including all the poking and prodding and plastic cups—this was without a doubt the one I found most depressing and personally demeaning, whittling our pitch down to a twenty-word Hallmark card, my hopes for legacy now riding on a half-inch ad, tucked in among a dozen others just like it, a dozen desperate married couples all scuffling around the floor of some all-night Laundromat in Utica, stuck to the heel of an old man wheeling his clothes home at three o'clock in the morning.

⸻

But I guess that old man must have gotten around, because two calls did come in.

The first was from an older woman, calling on behalf of her daughter. She said her daughter was a nurse, late thirties, and that she had been raped on her way home from the hospital one night. She apparently hadn't considered abortion, but she didn't want to keep the baby, either. The selling point apparently was that they believed the assailant had been an Indian—an India-Indian. "Because you know," said the mother, "those Indians are very well educated."

The second call was from the would-be father, younger than me—working class and proud of it. He was offering us a twofer: the unborn child in his wife's womb—a girl—and their two-and-half-year-old son. Blond hair and blue eyes, he said. But he also made clear he wanted money, and not just cover-your-expenses-thanks-for-your-trouble money, but a real reward. "C'mon, you gotta figure, solves your problem just like that. Boom, you got a whole family."

His only other demand, and he wanted this in writing, was our assurance that we wouldn't use Ritalin on the boy, or any one of those drugs. He was insistent on this. "You don't pump him full of Valium or whatever just because he's playing Tarzan in the living room."

I read him loud and clear. I actually kind of liked him. He was easy to talk to, but I was also getting a pretty clear picture that somewhere upstate someone's skull had gotten in the way of his pool cue, and he was looking for a nice lump sum and a couple of bus tickets to Florida.

I told him it sounded like he and his wife had only just started thinking about this, giving both their children away at once, and that maybe they should step back, take a breath. He might want to talk to her again, make sure she was still okay with it.

He said, "Now, I *know* you're from the city. Look, if you and I get together and strike a deal, all I have to do is tell my wife to sign on the line. She and I, we don't need to discuss."

I didn't press the matter. I did say that my wife and I would have to think about it, though. It was a Monday. He said, sure, he'd call back Wednesday.

He never did.

Women.

CHAPTER NINE

RUSSIA!

So, to review: In the spring of 2004 Elizabeth and I were midway through the seventh year of our marriage; six years into an effort which as yet had yielded one miscarriage. We were in the process of putting together paperwork for a second run at international adoption, the last attempt having been a complete waste of time. We had begun advertising in upstate weeklies for potential domestic adoption; we were in a modified stimulation cycle, meaning that I was injecting Elizabeth with drugs every morning just because, what the hell. We were beginning seriously to consider surrogacy, despite the fact that it can set you back upwards of eighty thousand dollars, and I'd made so little the previous year on screenwriting that I'd lost my health insurance. Our savings were gone and our combined credit card debt was hovering in the sixty grand range. I hadn't sold an idea in about four years. The book I was now committed to finishing was going to take five at least. And I had no publisher.

But you know, if all those thousands upon thousands upon thousands of hours I've spent watching sports on TV has taught me one thing—and I think maybe they have only taught me one thing—it's that you're never as good as you look when you're winning, and never as bad as you look when you're losing. So like any good team, we kept our noses to the various grindstones and just tried to do the little things right. I was very excited about my new book, for instance.

Here, I'll prove it.

1. The father of John the Baptist, Zechariah, was a member of an adopted Order of the Priesthood.

2. The people from whom Herod the Great hailed, the Idumeans, were only Jews by conquest, but who adopted their faith just as the faith adopted them.

3. If one accepts that John was driven into the wilderness by Herod's Massacre of the Innocents, then John himself was likely adopted by a small tribe.

4. According to the tenets of Orthodox Christianity, Joseph was the adoptive father of Jesus.

5. Back before that same Orthodoxy snuffed out all dissent, there existed a school of thought that rejected the idea that Jesus was the "natural" son of God, begotten and not made, believing rather that he was literally adopted by God, and that the adoption ceremony took place at the river Jordan when John baptized him. Hence God's line: "This is my son, in whom I am well pleased."

6. Among John's most significant teachings was that the children of Israel should take no solace from their bloodline. "Think not to say within yourself that we have Abraham as our father. The Lord can raise up children of Abraham from these very stones."

On the even brighter side, though our hopes were now strewn among several different possibilities, it was definitely starting to look like the Russian venture was our best bet. The agency we'd found seemed to be for real, and our personal coordinator, a high-watt angel living down in parts south named Ronni, was a completely trustworthy breath of fresh air. We never actually met in person—not until afterward, anyway—but we were dealing with her pretty extensively by e-mail, where she made liberal use of the exclamation point, and on the phone, where she did likewise. She also once or twice made the mistake of mentioning that she was headed off to aerobics class, so whenever she wasn't dealing with us, I liked to think of her running out on stage in a fitness competition on ESPN 2, bouncing up and down, walking around on her hands. But all that energy made her a good and thorough taskmaster, shepherding us through the process in a way that our former lawyer never had, sending us paperwork and making sure our Home Study was in on time. More than ever before, it all felt very real, and like it actually might happen!

And the strange part was, if we'd been basing our decision solely on what we wanted—that is, without regard for the fears that had been sewn into us by agencies and lawyers—Russia was the first place we'd have gone. My interest in Lithuania had everything to do with its proximity to Russia. And when I learned that the Romanian language is actually a hybrid of Latin and Russian, I was suspiciously excited. Indeed, from a purely cultural standpoint, and after all the different corners of the world we had been considering, not only had I no reservation about our child possibly being of Russian heritage, I actually kind of considered it an honor.

To explain: This feeling was admittedly without fabric. My actual hands-on experience of Russia, or Russians, was practically nil. I had never been there. I had never had a close Russian friend or even a friend of Russian descent unless you count Jews. Nor is there even a trace of Russian blood flowing in my veins, at least that I know of. I have a vague memory of my father once worrying that he might be developing hemophilia, but that's about as close as we came. I am of basically northern European stock—principally Norwegian and English, with various smatterings of Dutch and Swiss and who-knows-what-else thrown in. For the sheer sense of primal connectedness I'm much more inclined to picture an old man in a sweater eating a bowl of soup than I am, say, howling Cossacks, or peasants doing the squat-kick. All of which is to say that my affinity for all things Rus is a taste I acquired over time, and almost completely as result of my cultural interests and influences.

Where it all began, I'm not exactly sure, though Peter's theme from *Peter and the Wolf* wouldn't be a bad guess. And being a writer, of course—a "novelist of ideas," no less—I owe an obvious and very happy debt to the tradition of Tolstoy, Dostoyevsky, Chekhov, Nabokov, and so forth. Whenever I need reminding of the fact that there is actually some virtue to my line of work, they are among the first I turn to.

In point of fact, however, I'm actually not that much of a fiction reader, and so whatever insight or enthusiasm I may bring to the whole question of Russia and Russians I principally have derived from music, as mentioned, and sports, of course. They are what taught me the truth, or the lie I like to think of as the truth.

Born in 1965, I am happily a little young to ever have regarded Russians as my mortal enemy. If I held anything against them, it had more to do with the 1972 Olympic gold medal basketball game than the nuclear missiles they had trained on my kitchen window. I suspect that Sylvester Stallone also may have played slightly too large a role in my thinking, but like most people of my generation, I tended as a youth to think of Russians as, well, you know, hapless victims of a spirit-trampling system, plucked from kindergartens and drilled endlessly until they became hollow-eyed, but no less conniving emblems of all that is wrong with Marxism, Leninism, Trotskyism, Stalinism . . . that sort of thing. No doubt that old Red Army team of Tretiak influenced my thinking, too. All that talk about the "system."

It wasn't until the Cold War really started to thaw in the mid-1980s and Russian players began trickling westward, lured by the hard currency of the NHL, that I discovered the real truth: that Russians were not, in fact, the highly disciplined, mistake-averse robots I'd come to love to hate. Quite the contrary: they were the flashiest, most imaginative, most brilliant, and completely irresponsible players I'd ever had the pleasure of watching; the best skaters, passers, and stick handlers, at least on open ice, their chief flaw the propensity for slick, high-risk maneuvers that often trapped their teammates and resulted in goals-against.

The prime example of the type of player I'm thinking of is a guy named Alexei Kovalev, which is hardly fair, he being but one man, and not all that typical of his fellow countrymen. Still, Lexei is the one who stands out as the shining beacon of a certain Russian insouciance, whereby the glare of his boneheadedness was outshone only by the gleam of his genius. I was a big fan of Lexei. His style was not my style, but when the Rangers traded him to the Pittsburgh Penguins (along with a healthy chunk of the team's goals-against average), a piece of my heart went too.

So he was, to me, an early clue into the deeper truth of this creature, the "Russian spirit," but I doubt his style would have held such resonance had I not discerned its echo in the other realm where I spend most of my ostensibly unconstructive time, listening to music.

I was around thirteen when I began to develop a pretty ravenous appetite for the stuff, and one of my first instincts, once it became clear to me that pop/rock alone was just not going to satisfy me, was to find out who the guy was who wrote *Peter and the Wolf* and see what else he'd been up to. I understood it was children's music, of course, but there was still something to those melodies, something so distinct and pretty, but kind of weird and irresistible, too—that A-minor in the fifth measure of Peter's theme may have been where I fell. I wanted more. So I went out and I got more, and I didn't like all of it at first, but for some strange reason I still felt it was my duty to hang in there, that patience and perseverance would be rewarded, so I kept feeding my ear, and over the years and decades, I guess you could say I adopted Prokofiev, the way you adopt a player on your favorite team, not because you necessarily think he's the greatest player who ever lived—only Bach is Bach—but there's just something about him,[3] something that you get, or that gets you.

In Prokofiev's case, a lot of things. The gift for simple, new, and indelible melody; the ability to break a line in the middle and fix it before it's done; maybe just that abiding sense of total mastery, rendered at the service of play. Hard to put into words, obviously. There was just something in the places he took me; knowing they're not places I'd ever have gotten on my own, but they still made perfect sense to me when I arrived. They made me smile. They made me laugh, as did all the characters I met there, that whole gallery of buffoons and princes, ash-can girls, monsters, and ingénues. They've turned out to be some of my best friends, really—reliable and surprising, handsome, funny, brash, spiky, grotesque, patently ridiculous, achingly beautiful; all very individual, but all cut from the same cloth. They all look a little like Peter. They've got his features, but they've got their own secrets, too, their own lives, and there's no question that the time I spent with them helped to open me and broaden me, and introduce me to countless other good friends of theirs (and enemies, too!)— those from the family of Shostakovich, and Scriabin, and all those

---

3   In my case, the Mets had a third baseman named Wayne Garrett, and boy, was he nothing to write home about: a .240 hitter and about as charismatic as a glass of milk. As I look back on it, it seems clear to me that my devotion was based largely on the fact that of all the New York Mets, he was the one I stood the best chance of growing up to look like. But Wayne had his virtues. He seemed very well mannered. He could pick it at third, had a strong arm, a very good eye at the plate, could work a walk in a crucial situation. He even sometimes hit lead-off for that 1973 NL champion team (which goes to show you how good their pitching was). "Red," his teammates called him, for the color of his hair, though it never looked so red to me. Maybe strawberry blond.

great Russian composers other than Tchaikovsky. Mussorgsky, of course, the original slovenly genius. Over the years, I developed a taste for the whole emotional palette—the high romanticism, the despair, bitter irony, the lyricism, and innate sense of dance, all spiced by that exotic dash, there to remind: These people really aren't European. They sit between the east and west, and absorb a lot from each.

So for all these reasons, all these characters—because of Mussorgsky and Alexei Kovalev, and Sergei Zubov, and Nicholas Roerich, and Nabokov and Tolstoy and Chekov and Nijinsky and Blavatsky and Eisenstein and Richter, but most of all because of Prokofiev—dear Sergei Sergeyevich—when Elizabeth and I finally set our sights on Russia, a little light went on inside.

Me and Russia, we'd had this date coming for a while.

―――

Okay, but here's the thing: Adopting a child from Russia is, from a purely nuts and bolts perspective, a colossal pain in the ass. Kafka wasn't kidding. The first thing you have to do is put together what is called your Russian Dossier, though that makes it sound a little too much like something Pierce Brosnan gets handed in the first thirty seconds of a movie. In fact, your dossier, once it has been fully assembled, deserves its own seat on an airplane. It includes all your paperwork—the Home Study, certificates of good conduct, fingerprints, financial checks, reference letters, tax forms, etcetera. I don't know how people with real jobs do it, for the amount of time you have to spend tooling around police plazas, courthouses, and embassies, basically all the best bomb targets in the city. And everything you submit needs to be signed. Everything that is signed needs to be notarized. Everything that's notarized has to be authenticated. Everything that is authenticated has to be apostilled (look it up). And most of that has to be updated every three months.

But the dossier is only part of the drill. Ronni of the Red Bull also put us on to a required online multimedia course for parents planning to adopt internationally. We started putting together a photo album of our families for any potential appearances in court, just so the judge could see all the relatives our child would have. We started a vaccine regimen for traveling abroad.

Very important, we hired a local pediatrician with international adoption expertise to be our stateside medical advisor for when information about prospective children started coming in. Especially if you're adopting from Eastern Bloc countries or Russia, they—the experts—put the fear of God into you about fetal alcohol syndrome (FAS), because those people east of the Oder do like the *wodka*, and because the range of conditions associated with FAS range from math-challenged to massive retardation. But forewarned is forearmed, so we enlisted the best in the biz— or the most successful, at any rate—Dr. Levinson. Truly, in the tri-state area, you cannot swing a dead cat and not hit a client of this woman, though few will ever have met her. Any and all information regarding potential adoptees can be transmitted to her by fax or e-mail so she can review and then render a diagnosis about the basic health risks of the child at question: medium, high, and "It's *your* life."

So granted, some parts of the process were more sobering than others, but we did get through it—and a tip of the cap here to Elizabeth, who did most of the work. I was permitted to absent-mindedly profess my way through much of it, redeeming myself at crucial moments by running the more grueling missions—a day-long jaunt out to the Queens County Clerk's Office, for instance, which I was happy to do, since I secretly kind of enjoy taking public transportation to unfamiliar places, just to see the system work.

And mostly it did. Finally it felt like we were moving in the right direction. The dossier was nearing completion, but we also knew enough not to get too excited. There still lurked in the back of our minds the fear that something could go wrong here too, so we went ahead and made our summer plans as if nothing were up. Elizabeth had been running a theater camp in June for the last couple years. She went ahead and started preparing for that. Then we figured we'd head out to the coast and visit family. No more sitting by the phone.

<hr>

We started hearing about actual children toward the end of the school year. We had let Ronni know what our basic priorities were—we wanted the child to be as young as possible, and prefer-ably as healthy as possible; boy or girl, we didn't care—so when-ever she got any information about a child that seemed like it might be a match, she let us know, the idea being that if we sounded interested and there was more material to share, then she would send it along by e-mail.

But this is a somewhat sensitive topic, since the amount of information that adoptive couples are permitted to see varies widely depending upon what country they're adopting from, the region of that country the child comes from, the agency they're using, and timing, of course, since all these rules are constantly changing. Depending upon the circumstances, you might get a brief medical evaluation, a photo, maybe a video if you're really lucky. In other cases, you might not be allowed to see anything up front. You're just supposed to fly over to the country on what is called a "blind trip," to pick up your referral there and hope for the best.

And I'm not even sure what the ideal system would be. In our case, the information we were getting was fairly limited, Russia being a big country with lots of different regions, and a tendency to chest its cards. But even if we'd gotten our hands on a video montage of these children, complete with soundtrack, I'm not sure we could have mindfully processed the information: being presented with the desperate circumstance of a helpless, often-times sick child, and trying to decide whether at long last this might be the son or daughter we had been waiting for. Again, we felt torn, wanting to protect ourselves from further heartbreak, but also not wanting to feel like selfish cowards for turning down a child just because it appeared that he or she might have some challenges to overcome. I just don't think the heart or the mind can do that math, especially when all you've got to look at, usu-ally, is a grainy photo the size of a postage stamp, and a woefully incomplete, (sometimes poorly) translated, and therefore poten-tially misleading medical evaluation.

The first we ever saw, for instance—and I think we only did see two or three—included a diagnosis of "perinatal encepha-lopathy." A quick Google revealed this to be just about the most horrifying thing you could tell a parent, at least in American medical parlance: high risk of cerebral palsy and mental retardation. On further review, however, we learned that Russian doctors use this term pretty liberally. In fact, about 95 percent of Russian orphans are diagnosed with some degree of PE, which may either be because Russian doctors have a different understanding of the term, or—as has been suggested and resoundingly denied—they are offering a blanket diagnosis for all the neediest children in order to free them up to non-Russian couples. Perfectly healthy children are not, generally speaking, made available to foreigners.

So this is tricky stuff. There is a lot you need to know, and a lot you need to learn, a lot you need to think about and weigh and intuit. In our case, the evaluations we were seeing all seemed to contain one or two glaring red flags: HIV, hepatitis C, extreme prematurity; heroin addiction in the mother (which turns out not to be so destructive, actually). We could hardly be blamed for balking. We thought so, anyway, though by the third pass, we could tell Ronni was getting a little concerned. She said that given the parameters we seemed to be operating by, it might be a longer wait than she'd first indicated. We said fine. Stuck to our guns, and the referrals did dwindle, but we didn't panic. We proceeded with our summer itinerary. We flew on out to the coast as soon as Elizabeth's theater camp was done, caught some Shakespeare up in Oregon, then headed down to where most of the family is based in California.

I set up an office for myself. The plan was to be there for around four weeks. Elizabeth was in fairly consistent phone contact with Ronni, but things did slow down. No names. No faces.

We made do. Saw movies, rented movies. There's a summer music festival nearby for prodigally gifted students from all around the world. An upcoming concert featured Prokofiev's, *Romeo and Juliet*. We bought some tickets. Elizabeth put in some quality time with her mother, and I worked on outlining the John book.

———

Two weeks in, Ronni called. Only I was home.

"Tomsk!" she blurted through the line. "I love Tomsk! Everybody loves Tomsk!"

Tomsk was the town the child was from. A boy, born in January. She wasn't allowed to say much more than that, but she said she had a good feeling about this one. She knew the agent from the region. Polina was her name, and she trusted her, and she said that Tomsk itself was the best. It was in Siberia, but not furthest Siberia. A university town. She said she'd sent several clients there over the years, and they all fell in love with it. The orphanages were top-notch, the people in general were healthier—there wasn't as much drug use or alcoholism as you'd find in the big cities—and so the orphans from the Tomsk region tended to have very little developmental delay. In fact, she said if she was ever to adopt again, it would definitely be from Tomsk!

This was all great, I said. I cleared my throat and thanked her. Great news. A boy?

A boy, she said, excited.

And young.

Young, yes.

I told her Elizabeth wasn't in, but that I'd speak to her as soon as I could and we'd get back to her.

I called Elizabeth at her mother's. When she got on the phone she said she'd known when the phone rang, "That's Brooks. Ronni called with a good referral."

I said yes, seemed like it. I repeated to her everything that Ronni had said about the boy and about the town, and that she'd sounded very positive, like this was the one we'd been waiting for. Of course, Elizabeth wanted to talk to Ronni herself, which was fair enough, so we hung up.

When Elizabeth came back that evening, she said she'd gotten the same reading, and we trusted Ronni, too. She knew our situation, and she knew that a year before we'd been in a very similar place—out in California, waiting on news about little babies from far away, little girls in Romania. We had seen pictures of them even, lying in cribs. We'd given them nicknames—the Princess and the Comedian. But then nothing—no meds, no trip. Where were they now? A year older, and still in those cribs, most likely.

Here there was less to look at, but Ronni was saying we could actually go. We could hold him—a boy, a healthy little boy. And from a good region, a good town, Tomsk. Tomsk! This was the green light, no? This was go.

We called Ronni first thing the following morning and told her yes, let's set up the trip.

———

Adoption turns out to be a little like Hollywood. What doesn't happen takes forever; what happens, happens fast. Ronni said that

Polina was coming to America in mid-August to visit her daughter, but that she definitely wanted to be there in Tomsk when we arrived, so everything got moved up. We should be ready to leave in a week, she said, so we happily cut our California visit short.

As I think I've mentioned, that little stretch of coastline is stinkin' with relatives, on both sides, all of whom had some sense of what we had been going through, so they were all excited, too. They knew. This could be it. Maybe Brooks and Elizabeth were finally going to climb out of the tar pit they've been stuck in.

"So then is this the one?" they wanted to know. "Is it for sure?"

We told them what we could. You never *know*. You never know anything in adoption, but the boy was there and it sounded like he was healthy.

"But what if he isn't?" they asked. "What if you go and find that something is wrong? Or something has changed? Is that possible?"

Well, anything's possible, we said, and it was true, those sorts of things do happen. We'd heard about couples who go and find that something isn't what they'd been led to expect, the child had taken a turn for the worse, or died, or the birth mother had re-entered the picture.

"And what happens then?"

What happened then was that they usually had to go get another referral, for another child.

"In the same place, you mean? From the same orphanage?"

We weren't so sure about that, but it didn't sound like it. It sounded like they usually had to go to another region, wherever the next referral happens to come from.

The conversations didn't last much longer after that. That's when the relatives would go silent, and a little pale. "Wow."

The night before we left California we attended the Prokofiev concert. Or I did. Elizabeth ate a bad sandwich that afternoon and had to bow out at the last second, but I went with my brother, his girlfriend, and another friend. Great stuff, no secret there. Man at the top of his game, and by "man," I mean, "Man."

The music did obligingly recede, though, for passages—to serve as a muted soundtrack to the rush of terror and excitement that it was now my job to tame. So unknown, all this. So crazy and blind.

The first fall after graduating college, my friend Nick and I had been living together out on Long Island, working on the book we'd hatched together in school—already gambling, I guess, but that was the time for it. We had gone into the city for a few days, I don't remember why, but we didn't have a car. We didn't even drive—city boys—so we left our bikes at the pick-up spot for city-bound buses, which was about five miles from where we were living. The bikes would be there waiting when we returned—that was the plan, anyway—and they were, but we had miscalculated the light. The days were getting shorter, and by the time the bus pulled in, night was falling fast. We could have called a cab, but we decided to hustle, see if we could beat the darkness home on pedals.

Not even close. Most of the ride is a straight shot on a two-lane road, lined on both sides by forest, no lights anywhere. We had made it about halfway back to the house when we were completely engulfed. I was leading, and for about five minutes there—or ten, who knows?—it really was just the two of us sailing through the black. The only visual there to guide us was the glowing white line on the road, smooth and slithering, then hashed, and then for certain stretches leaving off altogether, just tossing us out into the abyss, the air rushing by, and our two voices yelling. We were lucky we didn't break our necks, but it was still about the funnest ten minutes I've ever known.

The day after the concert, Elizabeth and I flew back to New York, and it was on that flight that I was finally moved to lift my pen and begin this, what you're reading now. That was the flight when the gremlins in my overhead light kept playing tricks on me.

We had given ourselves four work days to put together the last of the paperwork in New York. Update our fingerprints for the umpteenth time, get our visas from the Russian embassy, vaccines. There had been talk about our possibly being able to complete the whole adoption in one trip. Siberia was so far away, and what with Elizabeth still being on vacation, that would have been ideal, but Ronni said that Russia tends to slow down in August. Everyone goes down to the Black Sea, or Italy, so we would definitely have to go twice. This first trip would be to get the referral, to meet the boy, and if there were no problems, then we would return some time in the early fall to seal the deal in court.

Elizabeth wasn't too happy about this, the idea of meeting our son and then having to leave him there, half a world away. She asked if we could maybe stay nearby during the interim—if not Russia, then in Europe maybe—but Ronni said no. The Russians didn't like being rushed.

So we girded ourselves. We had a phone consult with Dr. Levinson, who armed us with a whole checklist of questions to ask when we got there, and behaviors to look for: Was he lifting his head from a prone position? Examining his hands? Reacting to sounds? She said that in addition to the medical evaluation, she'd want to see photos of him—one head-on, one three-quarters, one profile, preferably expressionless—and that she would send us stickers as well, to apply to his forehead before we photographed him. That way she could get a more accurate sense of his head size.

We exchanged e-mails with other couples who'd recently adopted from Russia, just for tips. They were all incredibly open and generous, and all offered the same basic advice. This was big. It wasn't necessarily going to be easy, but it was going to be great. Be ready, be rested, be open.

I got back into a running rhythm. Ever since we first started thinking about adoption, the dirty little secret I'd been keeping was how much I dreaded the trip itself. Not the purpose, obviously, but the sheer exertion of it, carrying all the bags to the far side of the world, a strange language, strange people, food, money, all to meet a child you do not know, adopt it, and then, as your first act alone together, take it on a nine-hour plane ride back home. Perhaps I was sweating the small stuff, but it all struck me, from a purely physical perspective, as being one of the more daunting obstacle courses humanly imaginable. Really, right up their with labor pains and gall stones.

So that's part of the reason I'd been running so much, just to be sure I was in good enough shape to deal with all that flying and jet-lag and lifting. I didn't want my predominant impression of the journey to be exhaustion.

That last week in New York I decided to run a kind of special, commemorative route in honor of the upcoming trip. Instead of following the loop east at the top end of the park, I cut left and climbed the steep hill beyond the duck pond. There is a small round green at its top. I'm betting it's the highest place in the whole park, an emerald lawn, encircled by a little running track, maybe a quarter of a mile around, that's all, but not that many people seem to know about it, and it has always struck me as possessing a kind of alien-landing-pad magic. I'd round the green three times, three golden rings to make a crown, then jog back down the hill, across the road and into the woods, over the bridge and through the thicket, then back onto the horse path again.

It really was a steeplechase, come to think of it. A lot of up and down.

PART THREE

THE TRIP

CHAPTER TEN

HIGHS AND LOWS

SERVICE DATE FROM TO DEPART ARRIVE

LUFTHANSA 26JUL NEW YORK NY MUNICH 820P 1010A
   LH 411 MONDAY JOHN F KENNEDY FRANZ J STRAUS 27JUL
V ECONOMY AIRCRAFT: AIRBUS INDUSTRIE A340-300
   SEATS 43A/43C CONFIRMED
   RESERVATION CONFIRMED

LUFTHANSA 27JUL MUNICH MOSCOW 1115A 410P
   LH 3194 TUESDAY FRANZ J STRAUS SHEREMETYEVO
   V ECONOMY AIRCRAFT: AIRBUS INDUSTRIE A321
   SEATS / CONFIRMED
   RESERVATION CONFIRMED

SCNDNVN 01AUG MOSCOW COPENHGN 345P 420P
   SK 735 SUNDAY SHEREMETYEVO CPNHGN APT
   Y ECONOMY AIRCRAFT: MCDONNELL DOUGLAS MD-80 ALL SE
   RESERVATION CONFIRMED

SCNDNVN 01AUG COPENHAGEN NEWARK NJ 750P 1005P
   SK 901 SUNDAY COPENHAGEN APT LIBERTY INTL
   Y ECONOMY AIRCRAFT: AIRBUS INDUSTRIE A340-300
   SEATS 15D/15E CONFIRMED
   RESERVATION CONFIRMED

RESERVATION NUMBER(S) LH/J5KRJ SK/RA874

$1329.00 TOTAL FARE PER PERSON\\

One of my major failings as a human is an apparent lack of wanderlust. I don't dislike traveling. I actually enjoy it a great deal, but between my work and the amount of time we spend visiting family, I just don't set aside much time for actual physical exploration. Prior to this Siberian trek, for instance, I had never been east of Budapest, much less to the far side of the world.

I did, however, write about it once. The better part of my second novel takes place on an imaginary floating island/continent called the Antipodes, so named because it is located on the far side of the world from the protagonist's home in Dayton, Ohio. It is in the Antipodes that our hero ultimately confronts his faith, his fate, and the spirit of his late son.

That in itself wouldn't be so unusual, I guess. What was a little unusual is that a month or so prior to the Siberian trip, I finally came to terms on a contract to adapt that book for screen. Most people will tell you that's a fool's errand, but in this case, the book was nearly ten years old. I had written a few screenplays in the meantime, so I kind of knew how they worked, and I was being paid.

So that was the folder I brought with me to Tomsk. Not that I expected to get much work done, but I can't go anywhere emptyhanded, and somehow it just seemed apt that I should be revisiting the Antipodes of my imagination at the same time that Elizabeth and I were discovering our Antipodes here on earth.

7/26–7/27—A travel day. A day of highs and lows. The highs, very high. Thirty-six thousand feet, I'm told, which always gets to me eventually. Either it's the height, the sense of physical and temporal suspension, or some drug the airlines pump into the air filtration system, but somewhere around hour three of any long flight, I enter an almost Jamesian state of bliss, though it's a little sappier than that. Perfectly average movies move me to tears. There was a memorable flight I took one time, NY to LA, during which *Something to Talk About* had me in the palm of its hand for two hours.

No such luck this time. *Dirty Dancing II* never quite hooked me, but the rest of the in-flight service more than made up the difference; it was all so cordial and civilized, Lufthansa. The food was four star. I had chicken with penne. Elizabeth, spare ribs and potatoes. German beer. Camembert. All followed by a flourless chocolate cake with whipped cream and a perfectly ripe strawberry; excellent cup of coffee. My sense of personal and universal well-being was through the roof.

———

The Munich airport is set out in the middle of the rolling green countryside. Just fields and small clusters of manicured homes, all with the same tiled roofs. Elizabeth was the one who put the impression into words:

"We suck."

Indeed. If there were a prize given for the country that looks most like the architectural model of itself, Germany wins. Woe to the tree branch that takes a wayward turn. Likewise, entering the airport itself was like stepping inside a photorealist painting, all glass and reflections, beautiful clean shops, and luggage carts that glide on air. I bided time in a toy shop, salivating in front of an ornate wooden marble track set that made the ones that my cousins and I grew up on look, well, Amish, which I think they were. Or Shaker. I made note of the brand's website. My son should have better than I did.

My mood started to grime up a bit at the gate, however. Smokers here, and of course, the exciting and slightly scary part was knowing that all around us now were real live Russians! I was like a kid at a petting zoo, not that I could be sure who were the Russians, who the Germans, and who were just like us, neither. There was a young woman sitting across from us—small, with mousy features, a button nose, thin bleached hair, and an exceptionally muscular gymnast's body. I was pretty sure she was Russian. The businessmen were a tougher call. They stood in clusters with their overnight bags, thinning cropped hair and bullish faces; one was off alone, muttering into his cell phone, too low for me to make out the language. But was that the sort of brow my son could look forward to? Or the paunch? The weary smile? Did he look more "Siberian"? Was there even such a thing anymore?

Maybe it was all those unanswered questions, maybe we just never got to altitude, but the second flight—Munich to Moscow— was a less ecstatic experience for me. They're not called airbuses for nothing. No movie. The food once again was chicken or beef, but somehow didn't have the zing of the dishes in our earlier flight. My body was tired of sitting, and of course we were drawing ever closer.

Moscow hosts three different airports. The one that we were flying into, Sheremetyevo, is not quite as shaming a sight as the Munich airport. A thick beard of birch trees splayed across a basically flat landscape.

On touching down, the passengers all pushed and shoved their way off. I wasn't sure what the rush was until we got to customs. It was an absolute cattle call—hot, overcrowded, unsupervised. As soon as we realized we were in a free-for-all, Elizabeth and I did our New York best to elbow our way to the front, all the while glancing about us, taking in the living, breathing, unbathed gene pool, from the nouveaux cutting in line over here, in their wraparound pink shades and Rasta hats, to the little old witchy ladies they might well become, also cutting in line over there.

Eventually we funneled through, got our visas stamped, and met our Moscow contact on the far side. Giorgi, representative of the Russian-side agency that managed the logistics of our entire journey, Tomsk as well as Moscow. Giorgi was to be our driver and translator in Moscow—early thirties, Georgian, polished bald pate and a hipster take-charge air. He hoisted our heaviest bags onto a cart and led us straight to a ticket window to buy tickets for tomorrow's flight to Tomsk, and what do you know, they turned out to be way more expensive than we'd been told. We didn't fight it. I wrote it off as a kind of initiation fee, an acclimatizing rip-off, and paid cash, which pretty well cleaned us out. Giorgi said we'd get better exchange rates in the city, so we hauled our luggage out to his car—a sooty 1992 BMW, but everything is a little sooty in Moscow. Emission standards don't seem to have worked their way east just yet. That was the overwhelming impression during that first ride, in fact—of just how noxious the air was. My innocent New York City lungs could hardly take it. My ears were literally ringing by the time we got to the city, which had the sad look of erstwhile dignity about it, as if your great-grandmother got her luggage mixed up with a Vegas showgirl; or a five-year-old has been let loose with a box of neon Colorforms stickers, and plastered them all over her handsome, somewhat grim facades. Casinos and slot machines seemed to be everywhere.

What with all the fumes, I couldn't take in much more than that. We made a quick stop at the Marriott Grand to replenish our cash supply, and Giorgi was trying to explain the exchange rate to us. He must have thought we were complete idiots. We were both looking at him like zombies. I could hardly hear a word. Elizabeth almost collapsed right there. We needed to get to our hotel.

The Ukraina, it was called—an enormous Gothic-spired edifice about two miles north of the Kremlin, one of seven buildings that crown the Moscow skyline with star-tipped spires, though the Ukraina stands alone where it is, overlarge and grim, like a stranded mammoth.

It was around six thirty local time by the time we checked in and Giorgi went on his way. We were both spent, so we decided to keep it simple: wash up, have dinner at the hotel, and call it a night.

There were five restaurants in the Ukraina. We checked out each one, then settled on the first we'd seen—the Art Bar— because it had people in it, and an outdoor vine-draped veranda overlooking a park, which was nice, but not as nice as you may be conjuring from the description. The vine-drape was plastic.

We took seats outside and waited—not all that patiently, not sure if anyone had seen us come in. After about five minutes, Elizabeth got up and was just about to hand-fetch some menus when our waiter popped around the corner, looking an awful lot like a young Dmitri Shostakovich—plump square face, thin mouth, owlish eyeglasses, close-cropped scrub-brush hair. He spoke English, but had a verbal tic that made him a little hard to understand. We asked if they took credit cards.

He pondered before answering, "Credit cards are . . . mmm-possible."

I didn't know if that meant *ummm*-possible or *immm*-possible. I asked again.

His answer the same, "Credits are mmm-possible."

We decided to take our chances, gave a nod, and he left us to our menus.

The choices were ample, maybe a little too, and we were both having trouble focusing. I saw they had Chicken Kiev, but for some reason got it in my head that Chicken Kiev was Coq au Vin, which is basically chicken prepared as if it were steak, in a thick red wine sauce. I'd had it recently and kind of resented it, and I was in the middle of explaining this to Elizabeth, that in my opinion Chicken Kiev (Coq au Vin, that is) was an inherently stupid, pretentious dish, when Dmitri returned for our orders.

Russian waiters don't divide the drink and the food orders, so you've got to be ready. We weren't. Not even close. Elizabeth, mistaking my mistaken criticism of Chicken Kiev (Coq au Vin) for interest, went ahead and ordered it. I, if I'd been in my right mind, would have asked for another minute, but I didn't. Instead I performed an epileptically wild-eyed scan of everything on the menu, came up blank, tried to get Dmitri to vouch for the borscht, but he wouldn't, so on his recommendation went with the Caesar salad.

Caesar salad. Can you believe it?

Drinks? he asked. We said water, please, which didn't go over well. No vodka, nothing? I tried to explain, we'd just come in from the airport, it had been a long flight, long day, we were very tired. He looked at us as if to say, "Right, so how about some vodka?" but let it be and left us.

I slumped. Chicken Kiev and Caesar salad. Our first night in Russia—Russia, for heaven's sakes, and look what we'd done. Chicken Kiev was going to be way too heavy and salty for Elizabeth's needs right now, and way too much like what we'd been served—twice—on Lufthansa.

The Caesar salad was even worse. I could see it already: skim milk poured over wilted lettuce and croutons, maybe a shake of Parmesan. And right off the bat I'd violated the first rule of ordering food in Moscow: no uncooked vegetables.

I started openly grousing. I didn't like the fact that Elizabeth had ordered a side of boiled potatoes either, not when she could have had ratatouille. Boiled potatoes. Just how they like it at the gulag, I'll bet.

Elizabeth, whose exhaustion found her in an unusually calm, what-me-worry mode, offered to go change our orders. I said no, it was too late. We'd blown it.

I was acting like a complete dick. What can I say? I was tired, but then it got worse. Dmitri returned a moment later with our sparkling water, and mentioned that our meal would be another half an hour.

Perfect, I thought. My parasites were going to take a half hour now—when all we'd wanted was a snack and our pillows.

Elizabeth suggested we order appetizers in the meantime. Caviar and pancakes. I said, fine, fuck it, whatever. She got up to go tell Dmitri, and I tried calming myself. Maybe the caviar would be good. Expensive but at least appropriate, celebratory. But then Elizabeth came back saying that for some weird reason the caviar was going to take just as long as the chicken, so she'd just asked for bread and apparently gotten Dmitri in trouble with his boss, who couldn't help noticing that this was now the second or third time that the woman from the table out on the balcony had gotten up to amend her order.

I was low. I felt defeated, and I said so, by way of fake apology: If we couldn't even order dinner at a hotel restaurant, how were we supposed to look at a child and know it was ours?

I don't remember if Elizabeth answered or not, but then it was strange. Resigned to wait in grim, despairing silence until the food we didn't want arrived, two notes of shaming grace: There was Dmitri with two plates. It hadn't been a half hour at all. Five minutes, tops. As soon as he set the first in front of Elizabeth, I realized: Chicken Kiev is not Coq au Vin. Chicken Kiev is Chicken Kiev, a much better order for the occasion; safe and exotic, local.[1]

Even more miraculous, there on my plate was not Cae*sar* salad, but sea*food* salad. Dmitri, God bless him, had misheard. Or I had. One or the other, it didn't matter. This was much better. This was exactly what I wanted, tasty, small, not too mayonnaise-y, and it

---

1   This actually turns out to be not true either: Chicken Kiev was apparently invented in New York City.

exposed me to far fewer uncooked vegetables than a Caesar salad would have.

Elizabeth and I both gobbled down our meals. Credit cards turned out to be mmmmm-*possible*! We tipped Dmitri generously in cash and would have named our first son after him if we'd gotten his real name, but Russian waiters don't wear tags.

———

Wednesday, 7/28—Neither Elizabeth nor I slept very well. Twin beds. I slept better, I think, but we were both up and awake at six forty-five, and first in line to get our complimentary breakfast, served cafeteria-style in a banquet hall that, like everything about the hotel (aside from the rooms) felt too big for its purpose; a better setting for a convention—or a party function—than tourism.

The hall was crowded, though, and the spread robust—eggs, ham, sausages, cereals, breads, fruit, yogurt, etc. Highlight: the blini, and coffee served alongside warm milk.

We met Giorgi at eight fifteen to check out and head for the airport. Our flight to Tomsk was scheduled for eleven fifteen. Giorgi and I talked politics. A little about schooling there in Moscow—Giorgi has a twelve-year-old daughter—then Chechnya, then Iraq.

At one point we were talking about the transition to free markets and democracy, a propos of Iraq, but also Russia. There had been an article about it in the *New York Times* a couple days before, but Giorgi's take was instructive. He said part of the problem was that the Russian people really didn't come from the same liberal and intellectual tradition that gave rise to democracy in the West. They didn't have their Lockes and Kants, and so all those rights and responsibilities we talk about—the truths we hold to be so self-evident—they don't. Their communal and feudal history taught them different lessons, and he told an interesting story to illustrate—a kind of Russian parable.

"Imagine Piotr and Boris get into a fight at the local tavern, and Piotr ends up killing Boris. Something must be done. The families appeal to the chief of the commune. Clearly Piotr must be punished: say, be sent away for twenty years of military service, which, given the endless string of wars under way, means that Piotr would more than likely never return.

"The problem is, Piotr is a hard worker with a strong back. His work benefits the commune, in addition to which he has seven children. If he is sent away to war, the commune will have to support his wife and children, which will be a burden.

"*Well, what about Yuri?* thinks the chief. Yuri wasn't in the fight, true, but he has no children, in addition to which he is weak and lazy. So what does the chief do about Piotr killing Boris? He goes to Yuri's mother and says, "What if we sent Yuri to the army?" Yuri's mother says, "Fine. He's weak. He's lazy. He has no children," so it is agreed. Yuri goes off to war.

"There," said Giorgi. "That is what democracy is up against in Russia." (*And why Lexei Kovalev keeps making drop passes at the blue line*, I thought. *Because this Yuri guy is the one who keeps getting benched.*)

———

We were flying out of a different airport than the one we'd flown in to, Domodedovo. Still not quite to a spic-and-span German standard, but I was definitely buoyed by the sight of the crowd inside. Those old communes may not have meted out much Western-style justice, but they did yield up handsome crop of people. I was focused mainly on the women, but when we got to the baggage check-in, we found ourselves standing among about a dozen young men, all of a conspicuously sterling mold, most Aryan, but not all. Broad-shouldered, sleek able postures, they were wearing different tops—running jackets, sweatshirts, jerseys—but they all had on the same long black shorts, all wore sandals, and all smelled faintly of a morning workout.

They were athletes—the two older men milling among them, trainers. My first thought was that they were a college soccer team, as a couple of them couldn't have been more than eighteen, yet as I looked around at them more closely, I thought again. There were others who were clearly mid- to late twenties, and they had that *je ne sais quoi* of professional athletes, how whenever you see them not in their given arena, they're almost like exotic animals— antelope by the watering hole—and these young men especially, with their slightly elongated snouts, the Slavic pull at the edge of the eyes, giving them that sleek look of ulterior purpose.

But the legs were the real giveaway. They weren't overly muscular. Not sculpted for show, but sculpted for purpose, by countless hours of running and drilling and running and drilling. The effect was more in tone than muscle—nothing false, nothing extraneous. These legs were high-end tools of the trade.

I could even tell which one was captain, now. Among the eldest, he could have been approaching thirty. He certainly had the shoulders to carry a team, and an air about him, a slight smile on his lips, a comfort in being watched, and looked to, and informed. His wife was traveling with the team, howlingly good-looking, as was their son, two years old.

I was very relaxed in their presence, and happy. Even after we got our bags checked and said good-bye to Giorgi, I felt safe somehow, passing through to the gate area. We had our captain.

There were others waiting as well, of course—the usual assortment of businessmen, students, milling about the open area. A young couple, man and wife, with a boy, maybe four. They were all on the small side, fine-featured and handsome, if a little mopey. The husband wearing a particularly sharp pair of elfin pointy-toed boots that seemed to be in fashion, and their son had inherited his parents' good looks and slight anemia.

To our left was another family of three, and they were any-thing but anemic. They were enormous, but not fat; just two very big-boned blond people who'd found each other and had a very round, very cute, very bald, and blue-eyed baby boy. I could see them all on the cover of a dangerous brochure.

I was still doing okay, though, taking comfort in the presence of the team, now somewhat dispersed, grazing on magazines and sports drinks. The trouble didn't start until the flight got delayed. No announcement was made, but about ten minutes after our boarding time had passed, a new departure time was posted. No big deal. Elizabeth guarded our luggage while I went and got myself a soda from the newsstand. There was one with a picture of what looked like grass on the label; it looked refreshing. I bought one. Awful. Mint. It tasted like fizzy medicine. I threw it out after about four sips, and when I got back to Elizabeth, she did that thing she likes to do: She went and mentioned the matter at hand.

Tomorrow.

Tomorrow we would be going to the orphanage and meeting the boy, the baby boy, the healthy baby boy from Tomsk whom we did not know, but who was waiting to be our son. Elizabeth was just checking in to see if we were ready.

"Are we?"

How does one respond? I wasn't sure what "ready" meant. Up to now, everything had been so abstract. Up to now, we had been the potential father and mother to every human being we passed on the street. Tomorrow it all boiled down to one real child. Was I ready?

"I guess we'll see," I said.

"No, but I mean ready to be honest," she said, "with each other."

I knew what she was talking about; she wasn't meaning to cast doubt. She was talking about the railroader incident, that time we almost moved into the apartment because we each thought it was what the other wanted. She was talking about meeting this boy and not just being clear with ourselves, but being clear with each other.

I said I'd try.

At around twelve ten, a good hour after we were supposed to have left, one of the airport personnel took the soccer captain aside for a word, and the rest of the team started gathering at the exit. It seemed like the plane was ready, so the rest of us all quietly followed on down a flight of stairs outside into an absolute furnace of a day. There we crammed into a bus on the tarmac, all standing. Elizabeth started complaining about her stomach. I wasn't feeling all that great myself, but didn't let on.

When we got to the plane, we all spilled off the bus to find we'd have to wait some more. The fuel truck had just arrived and there was a general air of uncertainty among the crew. The passengers all milled about on the tarmac, some taking shade beneath the plane itself. Elizabeth and I had been warned about Siberian Air; that its fleet wasn't exactly state of the art. And suddenly the presence of the soccer team seemed not so reassuring after all. I felt like I'd seen that headline. "Strikers go down over western Siberia"—and the sidebar, too: " 'Posh' Author Felled in Snakebit Bid for Fatherhood."

We waited there for about twenty minutes before one of the flight attendants descended the gangplank and approached the captain again. Whatever the problem was, it seemed to be fixed; the captain was satisfied. His wife and child led the way up and in, then the captain, his team, and finally the rest of us.

We'd probably have done better to stay outside. The temperature inside the cabin must have been ninety-five degrees, but all we could do was sit and wait, and sweat. Still no announcement of any kind.

No one seemed all that upset, though. The athletes were keeping to themselves up in first class, but the rest of us fanned ourselves with safety instruction cards, while the flight attendant passed out little wrapped candies on a tray. The guy across the aisle flagged her down and paid her for a can of beer that he drank in two gulps, crushed, and stuffed in the mesh pocket of the seat back.

I was not so forbearing. Sitting there, feeling a little nauseated, with sweat trickling down my back and into my pants while Elizabeth plaintively murmured "Munich" under her breath, I went to a very dark place, wondering how it had come to this, and had any couple ever gone through more, gone to such lengths for so long, only to wind up here, making this ridiculously epic journey, all on the absurd premise that this was where they were hiding our child. It all seemed so desperately contrived and tortured and absurd. The distance we'd traveled, the vastness of the planet we'd watched turn below us for the past two days, and all the people we'd seen along the way, it made the point pretty vividly: this wasn't about finding *our* child, as if it were some needle in the haystack, victim of a mischievous stork. Clearly this was about finding *a* child, any child, and *making* it our own. And if that's what we were doing, then why did we have to come so far? Why was I sitting in 100-degree heat on an airplane that looked like it had been last serviced in 1950, waiting to take me even farther from home, to Siberia, the farthest place on earth? Couldn't I just have stayed in New York and cut a deal with that guy with the pool cue, pumped his kids full of the Ritalin they clearly needed, and call it a day? The whole thing would have been laughable if I hadn't felt so much like puking.

But finally the plane came to life after about forty-five minutes. It trundled across the steamy flat-top, rattling and joggling like the Tom Joad's truck. As we picked up speed on the runway, the vibration only got worse, and by the time we actually started lifting off, the whole body of the plane began to shudder so violently that the plastic panel covering the light fixture in the center of the aisle actually sprung loose and swung down over our heads.

That kind of broke the tension for me, the sight of the flight attendant rushing up the aisle to reattach a piece of the plane. Also, the AC had kicked in, and that made a big difference. As soon as we reached altitude, my mood lightened again. I took out my books and notebooks. I'd brought J. L. Carr's *A Month in the Country*, and that was excellent. And I also wrote a little. I had to register something about all these highs and lows. Was this how it was going to be? Because I like to keep things pretty steady. Who hollers from the mountaintop shall be howling in the valley, I know that. But I felt like I had to remind myself, or break these feelings down a little, because this was getting ridiculous, and the hard part hadn't even begun.

The lows:, I wrote.

> *an acute awareness of the absurdity of the mission; a profound nagging sense that something is not right; that somewhere a brake has been left on; that you have started down a wayward path and there's no reason to think it will ever lead back to the paved road again.*

Not too bad.

> *The highs: marked by an ecstasy-like embrace (albeit silent and removed) of my fellow man, in which all conflict, all*

frustrations, all disappointments and perils and injustices seem eminently and immediately resolvable by the simple and open recognition of our core human goodness, our mutual reliance and interconnectedness. A condition in which those frustrations and disappointment seem silly and fictitious.

Yeah, gimme some of that.

And to conclude:

Misery dwells on what isn't. Contentment embraces what is

CHAPTER ELEVEN

TOMSK!

The Siberian landscape never quite rises to the level of what you'd call a mountain, or descends into a valley. It rolls, and in mid-July, from the height of a gradually descending airplane, it looks mossy almost, green and soft; its lakes like mirrors, or puddles just after a summer shower.

As we touched down, three small birds flew alongside our window like kerchiefs on a string, and the air was just as welcoming as we all emerged from the cabin. It was much cooler here. It was six o'clock. The sun had another five hours to descend, but the shadows were long, and the bugs, of which we'd been warned, were out but not oppressive. June apparently is their heyday.

The airport was undergoing some reconstruction, so we were met at the gate of a chain-link fence by our two hosts, Katya and Polina.

Katya was to be our translator. She introduced herself with a slight bow. Mid-thirties, straight blond shoulder-length hair, and attractive, though her manner was discreet at the outset, and deferential—her purpose here, to serve.

Polina was our chief agent in Tomsk. She was the one who'd been in contact with Ronni, and who'd helped move up our dates so that she could be here when we arrived. She spoke very little English, but her manner was still impressive and forceful. With a darker complexion than Katya, her looks showed more of the Asian influence. Her hair was short, a stylish dark red. I don't remember what she was wearing at that first meeting, but her outfits were unfailingly smart. In addition to facilitating foreign adoptions in the region, Polina is also a neurologist, and a woman who knows how to shop. She stood square and strong on greeting, and damn near hip-checked me out of the way for the heaviest of our bags. I insisted, but let her take my computer as a compromise.

On our way to the parking lot, I asked about the soccer team, just to break the ice. Katya confirmed that the team was in fact the Tomsk soccer team—yes, professional, but division III, and coming off a loss. Not a huge fan, she could not confirm the identity of the captain.

We met our driver in the parking lot, Ivan. Polina's husband, and right there worth the trip. But for his gentle blue eyes, he was thick and powerful in every detail. A flat-top crew-cut suggested military service somewhere in his past. Indeed, if Ivan were something other than a human, it would be a helmet; if his wrists were something other than wrists, they would be riveting guns; his hands, inadvertent bunny-crushers. I couldn't take my eyes off them. I thought, if I am ever trapped in a prison camp, I want Ivan on my team. Worse comes to worst, he can walk through a wall, and the rest of us can crawl free through his outline.

His charge was a 1995 Jeep Grand Cherokee, whose dashboard, like most Grand Cherokees I've known, had a hair-trigger impulse to inform its driver of any and all areas of concern with the vehicle, true and untrue. As we all piled in—Elizabeth, Katya, and me in the backseat—Ivan's dashboard was telling him he needed new window washer fluid. I doubted it. He seemed to as well. He pulled us out of the lot, heedless.

The road from the airport to Tomsk is a fairly straight shot, maybe six or seven miles lined most of the way by a dense forest of cedar and birch. Ivan and Polina carried the conversation, through Katya, and Katya got in her fair share as well. They were all three eager ambassadors of their hometown. Leaning back around their front seats, both Polina and Ivan explained, in Russian, something of the history of the place, though I have to admit I was a little distracted. Everything was so new, and Elizabeth had been reminding me about the importance of looking directly at whoever was speaking. There is a tendency not to when a translator is around. But what they were saying more or less jibed with what I'd learned from the Internet: Tomsk had been founded as a frontier trading post back in the early 1600s. It took its name from the river it straddles, the Tom, which took its name from Toma, daughter of a Tatar king. Following the emancipation of the serfs in 1861, the eastern regions all absorbed an influx of settlers, but Tomsk didn't forge its modern identity until a couple generations after that when the State University was built there. Five more separate universities soon followed, making Tomsk the undisputed Siberian capital of higher learning, and the home of more universities than anywhere else in Russia, save for Moscow and St. Petersburg. Not bad for a town with a population of 600,000.

And here it was. Just as the tree line to the left briefly opened to frame a giant war memorial—two large bronze figures dramatically posed before an eternal flame—we swung right onto what is essentially the Main Street of Tomsk, Lenin Way. Some years back, local officials tried renaming it University Way, but history and the status quo prevailed. Certainly the new name would have fit. For the next half mile or so, we speared one university after another—polytechnic, medical, State—all interspersed with various historic municipal buildings, parks, public fountains, and terraces, basking in the late afternoon sun. The sidewalks were teeming with students, and I'll admit it, come for the purpose we had, I was agog, a dog with his tongue hanging out the window. It didn't quite make sense. If ever a town looked capable of absorbing its own orphans, this one did. The only explanation I could come up with was the dreamiest imaginable: Gorgeous, whip-smart coeds getting maybe a little too close to their professors? Career-tracked world-beaters trying to put a bad decision behind them? Woohoooo, we'll take five!

Adding to the generally fulsome air of the place was the fact, as Katya informed us, that Tomsk was at that moment preparing for its four-hundredth anniversary celebration. Weeks away. State money had been poured in, and the town was taking the task seriously. As Elizabeth said later, it was a little like entering a Richard Scarry book. Everywhere you looked there was someone else in overalls and cap, climbing up ladders, painting trim, carrying lumber, mixing cement, hammers dangling from their pockets.

Just past a fountain park, Ivan turned off Lenin Way to take a side road. This was for parking purposes, as it turned out, but it gave us our first glimpse of the more distinctive local architecture. Down a narrow tree-lined street, we passed through a row of what looked like log cabin, gingerbread boarding houses, complete with cross-hatch corners, steep gabled roofs, and the most ornate carved window dressings this side of Disneyland. If you see these, you apparently know you are in Siberia, but as much care as had been put into the woodwork, painting seemed to be less of a priority, or even staining. They were all gray and a little tired-looking, giving them all a weird dissonant quality of rococo decrepitude. I couldn't quite tell if we were driving past homes, abandoned houses, or historical monuments, and the answer is, we may have been doing all three.

In any case, this two or three blocks' worth of dilapidated splendor led us around to the back entrance of our hotel, the Siber. Ideally located on the corner of Lenin Way, it was subsumed by a thick cloud of plaster dust. The inside was being remodeled for the birthday party.

We didn't mind. While Ivan stayed in the car (Ivan *always* stayed in the car) Polina and Katya helped us check in, once again wrestled me for the heavy bags, and escorted us up to the third floor—no elevators. We'd been given a small suite—entry area, sitting room, bedroom, two TVs. We pulled up chairs in the sitting room and had a brief meeting about what was to come.

Tomorrow was the day, after all. Let's not bury the lede here. Polina said his name was Ilya. She didn't give his last name, but she said he was doing very well. Six months old, but "Big," she said, in English. She puffed out her lips and then pointed directly at Elizabeth to indicate the resemblance was to her, at least in coloring. Elizabeth's veins flow with the blood of the Romance countries. She's not dark, but at least she tans. There was something very calming, very reassuring about Polina's saying it.

More reassuring was Ilya's medical evaluation. Polina didn't have it with her, but she said it was a clean bill of health, and I didn't question it. No hepatitis. No HIV. No apparent drug use in the mother. He was a healthy boy, she said.

We turned to the paperwork, ours, and there we did run into a glitch. We assumed that the most of our dossier had been sent already. All we'd brought with us were dribs and drabs, but apparently the rest hadn't arrived from Moscow. This did not strike me as that big a big deal; nothing a couple phone calls couldn't fix. But Elizabeth and Polina both showed a slight flair for the dramatic here. We cleared things up, but there were a couple moments there where it seemed to me like all three women were on the verge of tears, and I'm still not even exactly sure why. I guess we were all feeling a little fragile.

But happy. This was all going very well. There had been talk of our all having dinner together, but we were a little tired, so Katya and Polina walked us down to a little shop right next to the hotel—a convenience store that sold sausages. Polina insisted we buy some. Out of deference to her, we yielded; bought some water for Elizabeth and some dark chocolate for me.

As for dinner, Elizabeth and I decided to take it easy and just have a bite at the hotel. Polina had recommended a small restaurant on the first floor. A nice clean space, café style, with square tables and a large pull-down screen showing music videos, which normally I'd have found intrusive, but which I kind of welcomed here. About half the music was English; a lot of French as well, and I have a lurid fascination with non-American pop culture.

The waitress we would get to know fairly well, language or no. Tanya was in her early twenties, if that, petite, always dressed in a crisp white shirt, black worker slacks, burnished brunette hair, bangs, a pony tail, and a definite sparkle in her eye.

I ordered the herring and vegetables, which was served in a finely chopped mélange bound by sour cream. Elizabeth had the salmon, though it took her a while to admit that it was salmon. We split a beer, and compared notes for the first time. The place was a find. It was amazing. Those houses, and the people certainly were beautiful, and healthy, and pleasant.

"We should buy now," I said, "before they gays find out and drive up the prices."

Our plates were more or less clean—or mine was—by the time that the video loop started up again. We stuttered through an intensely awkward, blushing exchange with Tanya about the tip. We weren't sure how much we were supposed to leave, but erred on the side of ostentation, left something like five bucks, and headed upstairs for a pair of cold showers. It seems we had neglected to start up the water heater.

But that was fine. We weren't complaining. We were here. We were in one piece. We did not feel so far from home. And tomorrow was the day. Labor Day. The day we see our son.

CHAPTER TWELVE

ILYA

Thursday, 7/29—We both woke up early. I slept all right. The windows opened, so the air was good. The bed was good. The pillows were far and away the heaviest I've ever encountered. If the purpose was for theft protection, well done. I couldn't have made it half-way down the hall with these babies under my arms.

Elizabeth said she slept almost not all—three hours, tops—which was too bad. It was the sort of day you want to be at your best. On the other hand, if there were ever an occasion in which adrenalin could be trusted to get you through . . .

We went down and had our complimentary breakfast in the hotel café: a rather spare offering of blinis and berry syrup. Elizabeth ordered more, and ate less, which again was too bad. Not only was she not sleeping very well, she was not eating.

It was still early, so we returned to the room to await the phone call from Katya. The plan had been for Ivan and Katya to come pick us up at ten thirty. Katya called at ten fifteen and said let's make it eleven, so I decided to go for a walk. We needed mouthwash and I also wanted to get a better outlet adapter than the piece of crap we brought for our battery charger. Remember, one of our chief responsibilities today—in addition to meeting the heir—was going to be photographing him and sending those pictures back to Dr. Levinson in New York so she could give him her medical seal of approval. I didn't doubt she would, based upon the things that Polina had been saying, but still, we wanted to be sure we were battery ready. And that we could get access to the Internet, which we couldn't get in our rooms.

So a quick stroll. The people on the street were a bit less comely than those we'd seen last night, basically I think because I was headed *away* from the universities. These weren't students, just people waiting for the bus to go to work, a little older, a little grumpier, a little less enthused about the future.

I did my best to blend in, walked maybe four blocks toward the downtown district, but still felt like a stranger in a strange land, mostly on account of that damned Cyrillic alphabet. Far more than the language, the electrical outlets or the elfin-tipped shoes, it was that alphabet, with all of its crossed-out o's and pi signs, that made me feel like I was in some kind of alternate universe, where everyone more or less looked like me, acted like me, dressed like me, but where all the ads on the street and signs in the store windows might as well have read: "You are on the far side of the wormhole. Return to the ship immediately."

Intrepidly, I did check out a local post office for potential Internet use. Nope. I passed a couple shops that might sell adapters but weren't open yet, so I popped into a small convenience store and purchased some Oral-B mouthwash. The store guard was very young. He hardly had his man whiskers yet, but I'm pretty sure he spotted me as a foreigner. I wondered, when he sees someone like me—here—does he automatically know why I have come? And does he resent me for it? Or does he like me more?

I decided that was enough excitement for now, and headed back to the hotel, sans adapter. Elizabeth was just starting to get ready. Flossing and scrubbing and tweezing and such. I did the same. You'd have thought we were getting ready for a job interview for all the last-minute spit-shining that was going on. I'd picked out a sea-blue linen jacket for the occasion; Elizabeth, a floral wraparound Diane von Furstenberg-esque number.

Katya called up from the lobby at around eleven. She said Polina would not be joining us today. She had other commitments, but our first stop was to go pick up the final member of our team, Oksana, the attorney who was handling our case. She was over at the Ministry of Education with our referral—that is, the paperwork that legally attached us to Ilya, and granted us entrance at the orphanage.

When she saw Ivan's SUV, she descended the Ministry steps, holding up the papers in her hand—light brown hair, a round face and eyeglasses. If you'd asked me then, I'd have said she was around thirty-five years old, and single. In fact, she is a grandmother, and just as her looks belie her age, her manner— unassuming to the point of being even slightly librarian—stood guard to a tough, discerning, and sensitive mind. Another you'd want on your team, for code-cracking and last-second heroics.

The drive from the Ministry to the orphanage was quick. Maybe two minutes. We slid up to a modest one-story building on another shady, tree-lined street. We could see there was a small yard in back, but not much else. Most of the houses and buildings in Tomsk look unoccupied and slightly abandoned, but that may be because there are never any lights on anywhere that there don't need to be. Ever.

Ivan stayed in the car, while Katya and Oksana led us in. We ducked through a beaded side door directly into a kitchen area that smelled vaguely of herring and bleach. From there, we ascended a step or two to an unlit hall at the far end of which we could hear the children, but we were not permitted there. We ducked into an office halfway down the hall.

This was the office of Dr. Yuliya, head of the orphanage. Tall, with cropped red hair and cat-eye glasses, she was polite, professional, and entirely confidence-inspiring. She sat us down and while the nurses got Ilya ready, she went over the medical records.

Basically she confirmed everything Polina had said. He was very healthy. Nothing much was known about either biological parent, but she ran down a list of the various tests and measurements they'd run. EKGs, blood work, birth weight, head circumference—all the things that Dr. Levinson had suggested we ask about. Dr. Yuliya said his muscle tone had been a little off, but that they'd put him on a semi-weekly regimen of "vitamins and massage," and that so far he'd responded well. Maybe it was the translation—Katya was doing her best, while noting all the pertinent numbers and vaccinations—but it sounded almost as if they were talking about a developmentally deficient adult, as if the next item on the list was going to be, "no teeth." My diagnosis: no problem here he wasn't going to grow right out of.

Then came the knock on the door. He was here. A nurse entered with a small, swaddled boy in her arms.

Elizabeth and I were sitting together on a kind of big navy blue ottoman pushed up against the wall. I was nearest the door, so the nurse first offered him to me. He peered out from his little bonnet. Our eyes met, and the voice in my head said, "Really?"

No outcry. No objection. Just . . .

"Really. . . ?"

The nurse handed him over, *yes*. I took him.

I was surprised, is all. I guess not too surprisingly. When you've had basically nothing to go on for a month, some false impressions are bound to set in. And Polina, remember, had puffed up her cheeks imitating him. That, and whatever residual connotations still attached to the word "Siberia," had all contributed to my sense that Ilya was going to be a Big Boy—a clean-up hitting catcher.

In fact, he had very refined looks. Perhaps that's just another way of saying he was much more of an individual than I'd been expecting, but I was struck by what a handsome, evolved face he had. Not just a well child; a wise child. I lifted him high and on descent, he smiled.

I did it again. He smiled again.

And Polina had been right about the physical resemblance to Elizabeth. The hair was dark. The skin had a definite touch of olive. More striking, though, were his eyebrows. There is a distinctive shape to Elizabeth's, shared by several of her siblings and cousins. More handsome than pretty, the transition at the apex is kind of abrupt, like the turn of a ribbon. Ilya had the exact same thing going on, though the eyes they framed were more exotic. I've always been rather partial to Slavic features, but Ilya's eyes showed a slightly more Asian than Indo-European influence; that pleat at the edge pulled to a nearly Oriental length—though again, this only seemed to underline how much more particular he was, more himself, than the nondescript mush of a baby that had been hovering in my imagination. His looks and manner were quite refined, in fact. Asked to give it a name, I might have gone with "noble Pangaeic."

"Hunh," came the voice again, "a child from whom *I'll* be learning," and by that I did not mean all that Wordsworthian stuff—"wonder," "discovery," "innocence." I meant it seemed to me that this little boy might have it in him to make me finally understand electro-magnetism. Or good opening chess gambits. This one, he could advise me in any number of ways. He'd been here longer. Why, he might even follow in the Old Man's footsteps, wear a crimson scarf. I'd kind of let that one go. Here in a flash, the idea was restored. This boy would go wherever he wanted to. Harvard if Harvard was lucky.

I passed him over to Elizabeth and got to work on the diagnostic photographs, though these already seemed a formality. This boy suffered no ill effects of anything, no rickets, no FAS, diaper fungus, or PE. Still, we'd paid the lady, so Elizabeth dutifully put the stickers on his head. With quiet dignity, he submitted as I got down on my knees and pointed my lens at him. One head-on. One three-quarters. One profile. No flash necessary. He complied, without expression. We took the sticker off.

Elizabeth then set him down in the space where I'd been. She set him on his stomach. He rolled over. Oksana spoke his name from the far side of the room. He turned his head. He reacted to the light in the window. Really, he could hardly have put on a more thorough display of developmental acuity had Drs. Levinson and Spock both been standing there with whips, megaphones, and nipple-biscuits. He focused on his hands, staring at them for more than five seconds. He gurgled just to show he could communicate verbally as well. He was very peaceful. Very calm.

I said to Katya, "You've heard the expression, 'Old soul?'"

No, not in English anyway.

"It means 'someone who has been here many times before.'"

Politely she translated the observation for the doctor and Oksana.

I switched to the video camera. Again, less for diagnostic purposes than to record the moment. Mother with child. The end of one road, the beginning of another.

Elizabeth, I have perhaps been too slow in pointing out, is quite lovely. Slender figured, with a full crown of long brown hair that frames a face which, though none of the features taken separately answer to notions of classical beauty, do combine for an inarguably beautiful effect, thanks to very large, expressive eyes and a smile that could win most state fairs. It is the sort of face, in other words, which, for its sheer expressiveness, tends to be a big hit among little children. As a husband, I'll confess it's a little bit of a mixed blessing, always knowing exactly what your wife is feeling; there are moments I could do without, but to a six-month-old, one can imagine few things more pleasant than to be held and doted on by my wife. So Ilya was getting his first dose, and to all appearances it looked like he was having a gay old time. She bounced him on her knees. She lifted him up and down, up and down. She set him on her lap and poked his cheeks, which he seemed to like. She used his own hand to poke his cheeks. Also very funny. And all of this is on tape, because there I was, rather unlike myself, inauthenticating the moment with my camera—Heisenbergianly screwing it out of itself, but how could I not? Dr. Levinson was making me. I shot a minute or so. I let it rest. Shot another minute.

This was all a little awkward, too, because in addition to the camera, the whole scene was taking place in front of Katya and Oksana. Dr. Yuliya had excused herself, but there was still a certain stiltedness, having to perform our reactions. We continued asking questions.

He sounded a little congested. Was it possible he was suffering a little cold?

Yes.

Do we know anything about the birth father?

No.

And nothing about the mother's family?

No.

We knew the answers, but just to fill the air, just to give our mouths something to do while our hearts took in. Elizabeth passed him back to me for another round of up-and-down, let him feel a slightly firmer hand.

He began scratching his ear just as Dr. Yuliya returned.

"And he's got a nap coming up?" I said.

That's right, they nodded.

He rubbed his eyes, like a good boy. He did seem tired. Katya went to summon the nurse.

We could hear another young couple out in the hall, waiting to come into the office. They'd been brought their child already. It sounded like this was their second trip, the court date. The father was talking to one of the nurses, or maybe another doctor. "Every

Sunday morning," he was saying, speaking from an endearingly choked and nervous place in his throat, a false depth. ". . . Every Sunday morning, waffles and strawberries. And we all sit at the table. And this happens every Sunday morning. Waffles. That's how it is. That's how it's going to be. And strawberries . . ."

He must have repeated this bit five or six times before his wife finally stopped him. "Honey—why are you saying all of this?"

He didn't bother to answer *Because I'm freaking out*. We couldn't help laughing from behind the door, then Katya was back with the nurse. I handed Ilya back, and the young couple swept by us, a girl in the mother's arms.

A girl. I thought. *Hm. I thought they said girls were almost impossible*. And this one was blond. A little goofy-looking, though. Fine. We stepped out into the hall and said good-bye to Ilya—handsome, wise Ilya. The nurse took him on her shoulder. He looked back at us as she walked away. We waved. We'd see him after his nap.

It seemed like the next order of business was getting our photos to Dr. Levinson. Ivan drove us to a couple Internet cafés he knew about, but neither one was open, and we weren't too concerned about what Dr. Levinson was going to say. It was around noon, so we decided to head back to the hotel, maybe grab a bite and some shut-eye before our afternoon session with Ilya.

Obviously we needed to compare notes, too. We sat in the large plush chairs of our sitting room, and Elizabeth began—but oddly, it seemed to me.

She said she wanted to get her concerns out of the way first, or that's what it sounded like. "It just felt different," she said. "And I guess I need to talk about it."

I wasn't so surprised by her tone. This was what she had been getting at back at the Moscow airport, the importance of our being completely honest with each other and with ourselves. I just figured she was being conscientious.

"And I don't want it to sound like I don't want us to adopt him," she said. "I'm just saying . . . this isn't how I expected I would feel."

"Well, but that kind of goes without saying, don't you think?"

She granted, but she still seemed curiously solemn.

"I mean, we had basically nothing to go on," I said. "I'm sure we've both been making stuff up, imagining what it would be like, and then a real person, a real baby enters the room. I agree, he was different. . . ."

"But I'm not even saying it was him," she said. "It just felt like there was something in the way, or like I wasn't being open enough. I want to be more open, and I'm worried maybe it's because of everything we've been through . . . I don't know, that I've built up some kind of self-protective layer."

Again I tried to tell her not to be so hard on herself. It was a first meeting. There were ten million things to take in, and of course it was going to feel different. He was going to be different.

"But that there were a lot of similarities, too," I said. "Did you catch the eyebrows?"

She nodded. "He looks like my father."

"And how smart he was. I didn't see that coming. He was really rather dignified, don't you think?"

She agreed.

"He had a certain bearing. He's going to be very intelligent."

She nodded, most likely.

"And healthy."

Again, yes. She wasn't finding any fault with him, or anyone else. After all this, to be presented with that—we could hardly have asked for more.

Yet as I looked at her, I could feel my heart beginning to sink, and here might have been one of those times I could have done without Elizabeth's emotional translucence. Or maybe not. Maybe this was its shining moment, but I was starting to see now, this wasn't her being conscientious. She was struggling. She was scared.

"What?"

"I don't know." She took a deep breath. "I just really wanted to hold him and feel like he was ours . . . for his sake. He deserves that, but it just felt like there was something missing."

The room got awfully quiet then. It got quiet because Elizabeth was being brutally and insistently honest, so I had to adjust, because of course I knew very well what she was talking about. I'd known from the moment she brought it up, and she was right. There *had* been something missing. That first hour we spent with him, anyway. I'd just been so relieved at how healthy he was, how beautiful and self-same, I'd set it aside. Assumed it was to be assumed. There had been other people in the room, and it was the first time, and however distinct the sense had been—of there being a certain gap between us—I'd bridged it with the thought of Elizabeth, or the sight of her there, a mother at last, finally with a child of her own.

But back in the hotel room now, sitting in our giant plush

chairs, she was saying no, that's not what I had seen. I'd seen her play it, but not feel it, and I realized then how much of the relief I had been feeling was really about her, not his health, not his clear intelligence or his bearing. I knew because looking at her now, and the almost deathly stillness that settled in around her, I could feel all my relief dissolving.

"But there was always going to be a distance," I said. "That distance exists."

She didn't answer.

"I mean that distance exists with biological parents, too. Isn't that what post-partum depression is?"

She nodded. Sort of.

"I think we're just realizing he's real. He's him. He's not the thing we were imagining, which he was never going to be."

She nodded again. She didn't defend any of what she'd been saying, or implying. She let me speak, because she wanted me to help her here, to pull her through this, and so I spoke, and I don't even think I was answering her. I was just saying all the things I'd been thinking long before this—as if I'd been rehearsing for this moment, which I suppose I had.

"And there's bound to be ebbs and flows. That's life," I said. "There are going to be times we feel incredibly close to him—you will, or I will, we both will—and other times, who knows? You know, some parents are really great parents to two-year-olds, but maybe they're not so good with the eleven-year-old. I'm just saying, it's kind of silly to think we're going to fly all this way and be handed an infant, and just *know*."

Yes, she agreed. All true.

"And I also think we're both very hungry," I said. "I don't

think we should think about this too hard before we've eaten. We should get food, and maybe try to sleep. Should I go get that chicken they keep talking about?"

She nodded, but she still didn't look too happy.

"What?"

"Nothing," she said. "I'm not saying no. I'm not saying we're not adopting him. I'm saying I want to find a way to get past this."

I agreed. "We should eat."

We went down to get some lunch. There was an alley that runs right next to the hotel. No car traffic, just small shops and farmers' stands, flower stalls. The sun was glaring down, and we were both feeling deflated. We found the chicken stand, and had to pantomime for the woman how much chicken we wanted—a half. I cleaved myself down the middle. Elizabeth pointed at her own leg. She bought some water and I got a Coke. The chicken came in a brown paper bag with some flatbread, that was all. No paper plate.

Back in the room, we cleared off the table in the sitting room, pulled it to the center, and set the chicken between us on the bag. There were forks and knives in one of the cabinets, but we dug in with our fingers like Henry VIII, quietly prying the flesh from the bone, praying for the food to do its trick and fill us up, because I was feeling awfully hollow all of a sudden, and raw, like we'd both been crying, even though we hadn't.

And I composed while we ate. I wanted to find some better answer for her because I could tell she was trying, but her mood wasn't lifting. The chicken was good, though. Rotisserie. And the Coke did start to pick me up a little.

This will be fine, I thought. We simply had to say these things.

We had to have this discussion. We needed to get our fears out of the way, and we'd go back, and he'd blow us away. How could he not? He was perfect.

"Because it's like John," I said, apparently having devoured enough greasy meat to speak again. I was referring to John the Baptist, because it seemed to me like what we were feeling was perfectly obvious, was simply reality, and it was reminding me of one of the things that had drawn me to John's story, something I'd never really bought about it, which was that scene at the Jordan when Jesus first appears—this man that John has apparently been preaching about, warning the people about, promising them.

"It's the same damned thing," I said. "You can't tell me, after all that waiting, all that expecting—believing that there is this One, this savior—that when this bearded guy comes walking down the banks, you just know. That the clouds part and a dove flies down? That's no good. That's not true. That's a hallmark card.

"What's true," I said, "what makes me actually believe the whole story is the prison scene," which I didn't have to explain because Elizabeth was somewhat familiar with my spiel, but I was referring to a brief scene after John's arrest. John's followers have come to see him in prison, and tell him what Jesus has been up to in Galilee. When John hears, he expresses doubt. He asks them to return to Jesus and ask him if he really is the one, or should they wait for another.

"That's the stuff," I said. "To that I say, 'Amen.' Because that's the point. You can't always be sure, but that's okay because he said so at the river. Faith isn't something you inherit; it's not even something you feel. It's something you have to *do*."

I was standing now.

"And that's all we're finding out here. We have to do it. We have to be with him and show it, and then what does it matter if we had doubts? Doubts are normal. They're going to happen now, or two weeks from now, or two months. The point isn't always *knowing*. The point is putting in the time and the effort, and that's going to be easy. This is a beautiful boy. This is an incredible boy, and we're blessed and so let's go back there and see him and start loving the socks off him."

She looked up at me. She wasn't arguing. Rah-rah team.

I had one more bite of that chicken, downed the rest of my Cok, threw my jacket back on, and grabbed the camera.

———

We'd already decided that for our afternoon session we would take Ilya out to the yard area behind the orphanage, so the nurses took a little longer getting him ready. We sat waiting for him in Dr. Yuliya's office, and I can't say I was feeling all that great. If I'd managed to rally Elizabeth with my little speech back at the hotel, I hadn't done such a bang-up job on myself. The whole ride over, I felt like I had swallowed a pit.

When they finally brought him out, he was in a frilly white bonnet. The nurse said he was a little more congested that he'd been in the morning.

Maybe the air would do him good, suggested Katya.

It was still sunny out. The yard in back was maybe an eighth acre of patchy crab grass, some half-buried tires, a gazebo, and a larger lean-to type structure they seemed to be using for hanging laundry. There were no other children; no orphans at least. Over one of the fences, there was a pair of teenage boys in the brush shooting a tree-stump with BBs, and every so often a stray nurse came out for a smoke. Otherwise it was just us and Katya, who gave us our privacy by staying inside the gazebo.

I was holding Ilya, walking him slowly from site to site. He did seem a little more subdued than in the morning. In part this was the chest cold, but also I think it was the sheer explosion of sensory data. It was a breezy day. The poplars were shifting, and Ilya's eyes were fixed on the dappling effect of lights and darks.

We stopped a while at a sitting post to let him take it in. I looked down at him, his handsome little face, those dashing dark eyes, and I was begging myself, yearning for something to catch fire in me—but far from it; that's where I went completely empty. Sitting there with him in my arms, all the little cracks of doubt that Elizabeth's admission had opened in me started turning into large, leaking fissures.

I fought it. I offered him my hand. He took it. He traced my palm with his little finger.

I felt nothing.

I told myself not to be this way, not to analyze my feelings before I could have them. I told myself all the same things I'd said at lunch. No moment could stand up to the pressure we had brought to bear upon this one. Clouds don't part. Doves don't fly down. Relax. This is nothing but cold feet.

But it felt worse than that. What was this feeling? I looked at him again, the fine peach fuzz on his forehead and his upper lip, while he studied my open hand in front of him—and aversion isn't quite the right word. He was too fine a boy, and I liked him—of course I did. That was the problem. I liked him fine, and I could care for him, no question. If this boy's parents had been good friends of ours and they'd died in a car crash, I would take him in, and feed him, and clothe him, and play catch with him and do all those things, no hard feelings, no regrets. But in my arms right now, that's exactly how he felt—accidental. It was actually physically jarring, the lack of warmth I was feeling. It didn't seem possible, after everything we'd been through—all those needles, and limo rides, and tears; after all that waiting and hoping and feeling like we'd been living in a desert, and then taking the flying leap of faith, saying yes, whatever you say; coming here and being rewarded with this, this beautiful baby boy, the most lovable thing in all the world, innocent and helpless and in need, and feel this? *Bored?* Because that is what I felt, once you stripped away the panic and the guilt and the confusion. He was here in my arms and I wanted it to be over. Sooner. I didn't care.

I kept fighting. I had to, because I knew—there was still no question what had to happen here. We were taking this boy home and making a life for him, and it would be a good life. I knew we could, and I knew we should. We couldn't come all this way and turn aside at the last moment just because we got scared, or because our feelings didn't measure up; we'd hardly slept or eaten, and this was just the first day. No reason to panic, no reason to be anything but joyful. I knew that, but I also knew that if another couple had come out of the orphanage at that very moment and said, "It's all right, we'll take him, we want him," I wouldn't have objected. I'd have said fine.

"And we just *knew*." That's what adoptive parents say—go online and see, or talk to one on the phone. "We just *knew*, the moment we saw him. Somehow it was meant to be."

That's all we'd been asking for, all we had been praying for the last however many years—not for a blond, not a boy, not a girl, not twins—just to *know*, to feel in our hearts that what we were doing was right. We'd have raised chinchilla if we'd felt in our hearts it was right. But looking down at this little boy in my lap, I felt like all I had was reasons—the same stuff that had been going on in my head for six years; reasons and wise counsel: *No, this is correct, do this, trust me, this will pay off in time, count your blessings and remember, nothing good comes easy, you just have to commit, be patient.* All the same frontal-lobe junk we'd been using since this started, deciding whether to do the Clomid again, or IVF, go with the Lupron or donor egg, or maybe it's time to start thinking about adoption, so let's use this lawyer, no, that lawyer, but stick with the publisher, stick with the publisher, they're the best, don't be an idiot—the same antiseptic, fear-based crap that had failed us every step of the way, when all I'd wanted was to feel it and know. The boy was in my arms, we'd taken the leap. I was out above the chasm, now give me something, show me a sign. I was begging, but if there was any sign at all, it was that they'd moved the far cliff back a few paces so I'd better grow wings fast, because I was literally hours from calling this boy my son.

I looked at Elizabeth. I had to believe she was doing better than me, but I didn't know. I was too wrapped up in my little green cloud. What I was mainly thinking about was, *How much of this will I be sharing with her?*

I felt sick, like something was seizing in me, literally dying in me right there, and looking back, I think I know what it was—the one thing that hadn't died yet, even after all those years, that little flame that never quite went out: Hope.

We were with him for about an hour. I took a dozen more pictures of him in Elizabeth's lap, looking down at her hands, and up into the trees. We strolled the length of the yard and back again. We started in the gazebo. We ended in the gazebo.

The nurses came out and cleared their throats. We handed him over. I don't even remember which one of us.

———

We still hadn't yet e-mailed our diagnostic photos to Dr. Levinson back in New York, so Ivan drove us back to one of the Internet cafés we'd tried before. It was open this time, down in the basement of the State University main building.

Thirty-three rubles—about three dollars—bought us half an hour. The computer stations were down the hall in a typically airless room, filled with about a dozen students, all male, and most of them with headphones on to muffle the sounds of carnage that their cyber search-and-destroy missions were meting out, their virtual selves all ducking around corners and blowing away predators, or thugs, or cops. The room smelled faintly of BO.

With some help from one of the room monitors, we managed to get the photos sent. Between the morning and the afternoon session, I'd taken about twenty, and we included all of Ilya's medical information as well. Busy work. I knew very well that Dr. Levinson would give the thumbs up, but at least it gave my brain a break, a buffer zone to help process whatever had just happened. I still didn't know how much I was going to share with Elizabeth. What does the strong man do? And how about the coward? Keep silent, work it through myself, gut it out? Or give her a chance to pull me through and risk dragging her right down here with me?

When we finally got back to the hotel room we were, as ever, tired, but we knew we should eat. Elizabeth hadn't had as much of the chicken as I had. If we napped now, that would mean a late dinner, and who were we kidding? We needed to talk.

We decided to head to the downtown district, near where I'd gone that morning to buy our mouthwash. There were some parks and theaters—broad spaces and buildings, laid out in the more expansive Soviet style. From there we could get to the river, so that's what we aimed for. We didn't say much on the way.

We finally stopped at a wide-open esplanade high above the water. The Tom River is pretty broad, maybe a half mile from bank to bank, and a stiff breeze was sweeping across. If we'd wanted to, we could have followed a ziggurat-type path down to the bank, but we decided to stay up high. There was a scattering of people there with us, taking in the view—parents with children, strolling girlfriends eating ice cream cones, old women selling little cups of black cedar nuts.

We sat down on the concrete ledge and that's where I tried to lay it out, what I'd just experienced back at the orphanage. But it wasn't easy making her see. The last she'd heard me say, I was charging us out the door of our hotel room—go team, go. She had no reason to think I wasn't still there, and in fact, everything I'd said at lunch still had merit. We had given birth today. The thing, the child, was Other than us, and we were saddened by this, and a little stunned, but that was no reason to be stupid and turn away. Perhaps this would simply take time. Most good things do.

I asked her, "If we suddenly found out we couldn't take him home, hypothetically, does that fill you with relief or horror?"

She didn't really answer. She thought I was playing devil's advocate, respecting the doubts she'd expressed this morning by quizzing them. It took her a while to realize our roles had reversed, that I was the one asking her to help me out now, and that may explain why the conversation moved so slowly and deliberately. It was all achingly long, wind-throttled silences, pregnant with thought. We didn't want to lose perspective here. We didn't want to misunderstand. But finally I think we both began to see, neither of us had done very well out there in the orphanage yard. She had tried, but she was still in the exact same place she'd been this morning, feeling closed and confused, and now I was down there with her. Something just did not feel right. All of which meant that here, on the cusp of finally being able to call ourselves parents—just a simple nod and all those years would be behind us—the question was back on the table. Could we? Should we? And the arguments for and against were more evenly balanced than I could in my worst nightmare have conceived:

Should we try to learn from our experience, recognize that all expectation is false and corrosive, and that to find love we simply had to open ourselves up and embrace it, not be scared, just do it, even if that meant committing the rest of our lives to a child toward whom neither of us had as yet felt a flicker of parental love?

Or should we listen to that voice saying no? Saying I don't

care how far we've come. I don't care how much we have been through, or how many people back home are waiting for us to come back happy. I did not come this far to feel this way. This is not how this goes.

It was a tough call, and we had to make it tonight.

———

We also had to figure out where we were going to eat dinner. Neither of us was particularly hungry, but we needed something.

Katya had recommended an English-style pub, but that was too far away. We found a restaurant on a side street away from all the exhaust of Lenin Way. It had an interior courtyard, medieval theme. The waitresses were dressed in Greek ethnic, with lace boots, calf high. There was a fountain and an open grill in the middle. And there was a photo album of the dishes. The one drawback was a very loud disco band playing in one of the interior rooms—a wedding band without a wedding—but that was no reason to leave. You can walk a long time in Russia looking for restaurants where the music isn't too loud.

We took a table in the courtyard. Service was prompt, as usual, but language was a problem, even with the photo album. The manager had to come out and help translate our orders: Elizabeth wanted a chicken and rice dish. I went with sturgeon, and another kind of rice. We both had beer.

As soon as our glasses arrived, we were joined by a large persistent mosquito.

I posed the hypothetical again, "So if I said we'd already

decided—that we were not accepting the referral—does that fill you with more relief or dread?"

She thought about—knowing this time that she was talking to someone who wasn't sure himself. Finally she answered: "Dread."

Good, I thought. A lead. "Why?"

She thought again, but not as long. "Because I'd feel like we'd been handed this gift and hadn't even been able to see it." She started crying, pretty hard.

I took her hand. That was a good answer. That meant we had been blessed, didn't it? That meant we should try to see it.

But no, it didn't. We hadn't seen it, and we couldn't. That was her point. And I think I probably started crying too. We were a mess.

Elizabeth was still weeping when the food came.

And again, I can't say as I remember much of what was said, as I'm not sure that much was said, what with the food, the loud music, the mosquito buzzing around our beer glasses. I know that midway through the meal, we were still at a loss, because Elizabeth made a kind of prediction. She said that even though she still had no idea what we were going to decide, she felt certain that some day we were going to look back on this moment, and we would know that it was the hardest decision we had ever had to make, but we would also know why we made it. She sounded pretty convinced.

I could only nod. I hoped she was right, but without knowing what the decision was. . . .

So I'm not even sure where the shift occurred, or if it had happened already, back in the yard when Ilya took my hand, or sitting by the river, or just taking one more sip of beer, because I don't think either of us ever said it out loud or shook on it. I just think it finally just became obvious that if we both really felt this way, it didn't need to be said.

We barely touched our food. My sturgeon was actually pretty revolting. Elizabeth's chicken seemed better, but she hardly touched it. When we asked for the check, the manager came out to ask why we hadn't eaten. He was being playful, but there does seem to be a pretty strong expectation among Russians that you clean your plate. We told him it wasn't the food, we were having a moment. The whole place knew we were having a moment, and they'd all been very nice about it, the waitresses and the people at the other tables. We apologized and left a big tip, and started the walk back to the hotel, pretty much the two most devastated people on earth.

But oddly the earth didn't seem like a very big place that night. The moon was up. I could feel our families out there, and all our friends a half a world away, putting in their prayers for us, wondering how we were doing and being all excited for us. I thought of how sad they were going to be when they found out, and confused, even though to me there seemed something awfully inevitable about what had happened here today. After all the dead-end roads we'd taken over the years, and all the culprits we'd been led to suspect—our bodies, our doctors, lawyers, foreign bureaucrats—finally it had come to this. We'd been handed a child. All we'd had to do was say yes and all of that pain would have been behind us. We would be parents. But we still couldn't bring ourselves, and we had no one or nothing to blame but us, and something in us saying no, this isn't right.

When we got back to the room, I turned on my computer and

together we looked at all the photos I'd taken of Ilya that day. We clicked through them like a slide show: Ilya in Dr. Yuliya's office, in Elizabeth's lap, and outside in his bonnet, looking up at all the leaves. I didn't say anything until we'd seen the last.

"Change your mind?"

She shook her head.

Me neither.

We knew the first person we had to call was Ronni. She would be the one to get the ball rolling, but I was decked. I felt like I'd just pushed a piano up five flights of stairs, and I had fifty more to go.

Somehow Elizabeth was not, and I will until the end of my days stand in awe of her performance that evening. While I staggered through the suite door and collapsed on the bed, all eight hundred pounds of me, Elizabeth—the world's oddest cobbling of lace and nails—picked up the phone.

She called her sister Anne first, out in California, just to drum up the resolve. I guess it was around six a.m. California time. Anne was home, and listened, and though I can't say as I paid very close attention—I was pre-verbal, lolling my head back and forth on the pillow—I could sense from Elizabeth's delivery that she was gaining in conviction.

"There just wasn't a connection . . ."

I'm not sure how long they were on. Maybe half an hour, but as soon as they were done, Elizabeth called Ronni. It was now around eight a.m. EST, and I could tell Ronni was stunned on the other end, but Elizabeth was being pretty forceful. She wasn't hearing opposition. "He didn't feel like our son . . . and I know, one of the things that makes it a little easier is knowing what a sweet little boy he is, and knowing that some other family is going to snap him up. But he just didn't feel like ours." All of which was true, but it was also yielding up a wave of consequences—I could practically hear the whir of Ronni's brain, calculating all the contingencies that would have to set in motion for us, getting back all our paperwork, flying back to Moscow, seeing if any other referrals had just come in—it pressed against my brain like a lead-lined quilt and sent me off to a cowardly cowardly sleep.

CHAPTER THIRTEEN

SERGEI

Friday, 7/30—I drifted awake pretty much as I had fallen asleep, to the sound of Elizabeth talking on the phone. She'd gotten up before me and was back on with Ronni again, going over what came next. Ronni had called Polina in the meantime; woke her up in the middle of the night to tell her we would not be adopting Ilya.

Polina had been a little stunned, according to Ronni, and not surprisingly. First there was Ilya to think of, but also I'm sure she felt she had gone out of her way to hand-pick this gorgeous child for the poor couple she'd been hearing about back in New York, and here we were turning up our noses. She'd told Ronni that the chances of getting another referral in Tomsk were slim to none, which meant that in all likelihood we would have to get our paperwork back from her, fly back to Moscow tomorrow, and check in with our agency there, to see if they'd found any referrals in another region. Ronni was already talking about another city about two hours south of Moscow, Saratov, but if there was nothing there, we might just be sent home.

When Elizabeth reported all this to me, I nodded, numb. This was pretty much what we expected, but it still felt a little like April Fool's to me. I couldn't imagine dredging up the energy it was going to take to make a whole new trip, fly to a new strange place, meet another little boy . . .

As soon as I'd brushed and combed, I called home. So far only Elizabeth's sister knew what had happened. I hadn't spoken to anyone stateside since we'd left.

My mother picked up, and as soon as she registered who it was on the other end of the line, her voice lit up: her son, calling from the far side of the world, a day after meeting the boy. She asked, "Have you seen him yet?"

I didn't beat around the bush. I said, "Yes. We met him yesterday. We were with him for about an hour in the morning and another hour in the afternoon, and he was very healthy boy, and very cute and charming," my voice began faltering, "but for some reason we just . . . it wasn't right, and we're not going to be adopting him."

I'm not sure I got the last part out. I'm not sure I could have, but she was also cutting me off. "You've done the right thing," she said, so quickly and readily that in retrospect I can't help wondering if deep down she'd already known there was something off. Here I was saying no, and there she was, seven thousand miles away, saying, *Yes, that's right. You're right.*

She launched in on an odd comparison to which I was only half listening. It had something to do with some friends she knew who decided not to move to Chicago because they were afraid of how the move would affect the children, and how that was a mistake because parents have to think of themselves first. They have to be comfortable and happy and at peace with their lives and their decisions, and if they are, the children will be happy and at peace as well. It did seem an odd comparison, but I didn't mind. All I wanted was to hear another voice saying, yes. Yes. Good. I trust you.

It was a great relief. I started crying.

"I wish I could help you through this," she said.

I told her she had, she was. I asked if she would repeat what she'd said to Elizabeth and handed over the phone, and started crying again.

———

Once we'd hung up and dried off, Elizabeth and I went down to have some breakfast in the café. No videos were playing, but the speakers were piping in Sting's greatest hits, a mid-eighties vintage I knew pretty well—"Seven Days," "I'm Mad About You," "If I Ever Lose My Faith." I'm no Sting loyalist, but this morning, just to hear a familiar voice, he was manna.

I ordered eggs. I'd learned that much, but the waitress was slow getting around to us, and someone somewhere had mentioned something about Russian waiters ignoring Americans. I had no idea. I was too busy trying to fathom the days ahead. And years. They splayed out before me, a tumbleweed wasteland.

I wasn't having second thoughts, though. It turns out there's a difference between doing something you desperately don't want to, and doing something you think you'll regret. That boy had not been our son. And I thought of what Elizabeth had been saying the night before to Ronni, and how true it was—that if Ilya hadn't been as impressive as he was, if he'd been sick or feeble or if there'd have been any doubt in our minds that some young couple out there was going to come to Tomsk, soon, look down at him and say "Thank God, thank God he's here," we could not have done what we were doing.

An image had taken form in my mind, of me holding Ilya on my lap and leaning over him, and there being literally a whole ocean above the two us, a great roiling sea of common sense and expectation pressing down on my back, pushing me down toward him, trying to get me to kiss him and call him son, but I couldn't. All I could do was keep him warm and dry until his true parents came and found him, and that was going to be a very happy, very blessed family.

So with that straw of consolation, all curiously played to the tune of "Moon Over Bourbon Street," we ate our eggs. I drank my cup of coffee; Elizabeth had her juice.

We got back up to the room in time for a call from Katya, who confirmed that Polina had been pretty dismayed by our decision, though she herself, Katya, professed sympathy: "I understand you very well." She said that Polina and Oksana and she would come meet us in the room in at eleven to go over what we should do next.

We still had an hour and a half. I flipped to the back of my journal and began drafting a letter to Polina, a formal act of contrition. Elizabeth read one of the two books she had to read for school, *The Giver* (which turns out to be about the sacrifice of children), but we were restless. As soon as I'd blocked in a serviceable draft, we decided we should get a real printout of the letter, something we could actually hand over to Polina.

That meant walking to the Internet café at the University,

about a mile up Lenin Way. It was a bright day, and an odd walk, I have to say. Thanks to my mother's unvarnished support, thanks to Elizabeth's sister Anne, thanks to the sun and eggs and coffee and Sting, as well as a growing determination that, however awful, what we were doing was not wrong, I wasn't actually feeling so low.

I was apparently feeling well enough, for instance, to indulge in a little people watching—which is not that hard to do in Tomsk. Not hard at all, as in fact, one of the more pleasant side-bars of our trip so far was just how good-looking the people were. Americans tend to think that wherever they go, I know, but I wasn't prepared for just how good-looking; or to be more specific, how good-looking the women were; to be even more specific, how good their bodies were; to be even more specific than that, how good their asses were. And believe me, I wouldn't risk squandering your pity by saying so, by admitting that right in the middle of this, my darkest hour, I was capable of enter-taining such a puerile interest—if it hadn't been so phenome-nally, spectacularly true, and Elizabeth will back me up on this. As far as I'm concerned, the whole Judeo-Christian concept of what makes a good ass might well have been born in Tomsk, Russia, and can be seen on full display between June and August, boogalooing down Lenin Way in mostly white slacks that could not be more form-fitting if they'd been applied with a can of spray paint. God bless those long winters, these people sure do strut when the sun comes out, and you can choose any metric you like—average, mean, median, toss our high and low scores, or just go with your best—it is a stunning overall effect. If these people knew the back-flips the rest of the world is doing over

Anna Kournikova, they'd be mystified. The woman would be a seven in Tomsk.

Anyway, so yes, I confess, that as we made our way down to the Internet café to write our letter of explanation to Polina, I was counting myself fortunate in the fact that I had only found this place now, as I was approaching forty and my testosterone levels were beginning to slip, because I swear to God if I'd come there was I was seventeen, I'd have died from saliva loss.

We did reach our destination, though. I screwed my head back on, we paid our thirty-three rubles, and descended to the room of unshowered warriors in their headphones. We sat side by side tweaking what I'd written. Half an hour later, the print-off read as follows:

Dear Polina,

Elizabeth and I both understand how confusing and mysterious the decision we've made must seem to you. It is confusing and mysterious to us as well, one of the most difficult decisions we have ever had to make, but it is based upon instincts that, for our sake as well as Ilya's, we did not feel we could ignore.

We want you to know how truly honored and humbled we are to have been offered the opportunity to come to Tomsk and meet all of you, and Ilya too. The work that you do—and Katya, and Ivan, and all the caregivers at the orphanage, and Ronni back in Florida—all trying to help these children and couples like us is selfless and extraordinary. Couples who came here before told us what a great town Tomsk is. Still, we could never have imagined finding such a beautiful landscape on the far side of the world, such a special town filled with such warm and

happy and handsome people. Nor could we have imagined being
presented such a beautiful, charming baby, whose smile and
health testify to the selfless work of all of you. We know and we
pray that he will bring joy and fulfillment to another family
very soon.

Please know that though we are saddened by our decision, we
will think of you and Tomsk with great affection, and we hope
that the orphanage will accept our gifts as an expression of
respect and gratitude. The children all deserve more, but it helps
knowing that they are in such capable, sensitive, and caring
hands.

Sincerely,
Brooks and Elizabeth Hansen

It was a good thing, writing that. It put our heads together, and in the right place, and just about exactly filled the time we needed to fill. We had to hustle to get back to the hotel in time. Elizabeth dressed in a white silk square-necked shirt and a floral print skirt, black on creamy white, worth mentioning only because when the women arrived—Katya, Oksana, and Polina— Polina was wearing the *exact* same outfit, but in negative—black silk shirt, same floral print skirt, but creamy white on black. Portent of good or ill, I couldn't tell. She was curt.

We took our places. Katya and Oksana shared one of the large easy chairs; Polina took the other. Elizabeth was on more of a dining room chair and I sat on the rolling ottoman. First order of business, we handed Katya the letter we'd written and asked if she'd read it aloud. She did, but quickly. I adored Katya, and of course I can't speak to how accurate a job she does at translating. I assume it's spotless, but I have to say her tone in this instance seemed a little off. She sounded like she was reminding us all about the rules of a card game.

Polina sat forward as she listened, nodding periodically. I thought we might have thawed her a little, but as soon as Katya had finished, Polina turned to us, very businesslike, pulling her skirt down over her knees and asked (through Katya):

"So how can we be sure that you're serious about continuing?"

A stern response, but give her credit, it was the only question worth asking, and I for one didn't really know the answer.

Elizabeth gave it a shot. "We understand we may need to consider children with greater medical risk."

Polina certainly agreed with that, but repeated what we'd already been told: that here in Tomsk, there was very little chance there'd be another referral. "Ninety-nine percent chance," she put it, "against."

We understood. Elizabeth told her we'd already spoken to Ronni and that she was calling the agency in Moscow to see if there were any referrals coming out of Saratov.

Polina shrugged. She didn't know about other regions. For now there was some paperwork to be done. Oksana had brought a form from the Ministry of Education that we needed to fill out and sign, stating that we were not adopting Ilya and giving the reason why.

This is where things got a little sticky. Ronni had warned Elizabeth about this, the fact that we would be called upon to justify our decision in writing, and Elizabeth and I had already discussed the matter briefly. The question was whether, instead of going into some mealy-mouthed attempt at describing something that basically defied explanation—and that as such might make us seem indecisive and incapable of actually committing—we might be better served by offering a more clear-cut, easy-to-understand reason. Ronni had wondered the same. Unfortunately, only two possibilities presented themselves, neither one very appealing: the first would have been the fear that Ilya might be suffering some sort of attachment disorder—which was complete bullshit, because if anyone here was suffering an attachment disorder, it was us. The second was that there might have been some confusion about his race. As I say, the referral has listed him as Caucasian, but there was reason to think this might not have been entirely true. The suggestion would have been that Elizabeth and I had grappled with this issue some years before—of whether we'd wanted to take on the challenge of being a family of mixed race—and ultimately decided against it. That's part of the reason we'd come to Russia.

Needless to say, neither of us was too crazy about this idea either. It was an obscene, not to say wholly misleading, reduction of an experience that had been far more complex and heart-rending. Imperfectly worded, it was going to make us sound like a pair of abject racists. Also, the truth was we really had no idea what Ilya's racial make-up was. He was four months old, for heaven's sake, and there was no record of his biological father. Whatever he was, it was an extremely subtle and accommodating blend, which both Elizabeth and I had actually found strangely moving. If I'd had to choose a name for it other than "noble Pangeaic," I might have gone with "mankind's salvation."

But I think what bothered me most of all is that I just hate the idea—I am principally opposed to the idea—of telling people what you think they'll understand; that is, reframing the truth to suit the perceived pin-headedness of the person you're dealing with. Jesus's parables notwithstanding, I think it's arrogant, dishonest, and doomed. I really really really think that's where all the trouble starts.

That said, I have to admit that in this instance, of literally having to fill in a blank on a page to be read by some technocrat in an underground cubicle, I did buy the logic. Just say we had our hearts set on a ruby, got handed a sapphire. Honest mistake.

To Elizabeth went the dubious honor of trotting out this idea. Katya dutifully translated, and Oksana even started writing it down on the form—she being the secretary of the event—but I could tell there wasn't a whole lot of enthusiasm in the room, especially coming from Polina, who sat rod-straight in the easy chair.

I moved to make sure they understood, as Elizabeth had as well: We were only suggesting this as a tack. This was *not* what we felt. I was frank. "Look, what we don't want is to write anything on that form that some judge might look at down the line and hold against us. So you tell us, do you think a judge would be inclined to accept this as an explanation? Do you think he would be sympathetic? Or she? To this?"

All three women shook their heads.

"Well, then cross it out." I said, "because it's not true. The truth," I said, now looking beseechingly at Katya, as one has to when invoking truth as a second resort, "the truth is that we simply . . . didn't feel any connection. We just didn't feel . . . that he was meant to be our son."

I tried to be more clear, but as you can imagine, it wasn't easy conveying what we had been going through for the last twelve hours, then having that siphoned from my flailing English into Katya's Russian—and all so that Oksana could whittle it down to a two-inch phrase and ink it in on an official government document that would forever linger the archives of the Tomsk Ministry of Education.

It was, in short, about as brutal a conversation as one could conceive, and it was hard to tell if they were hearing me. Polina's lips were a locked purse, Oksana's attention was divided between the form and the phone call she was making; she was actually on hold at the Ministry. Katya was still struggling just to understand me, squinting at my mouth, which was probably moving a little quickly, but I was trying to convey to them the fact that this had nothing to do with ethnicity or attachment disorders or anything you could put a finger on. It was about us and that boy—that stunning little boy—and the fact that when we had held in our arms, there was just something missing. The connection was not there.

Polina nodded, she understood it now. She said something to Katya, who translated: "So then we will write that you have no warmth in your hearts."

This is where Elizabeth burst into tears. "Nooo," she cried. "I *love* children!" She pretty much yelled this out loud at the room, loud enough for the neighboring guests to hear, and God too, and high time, if you ask me, because they all needed to hear it—the three women here, and God and all the gods and all the judges in Russia—that this was a woman whose struggle to achieve motherhood not only represented a personal tragedy of the first order, but a tragedy for children of the world as well. She had given her life to them, day in day out for the last eighteen years, caring for *other people's kids*, teaching them, protecting them, solving their problems. All she wanted was one of her own, but she'd been made to feel like a failure at that for the last six years, and now here we were sitting in a boiling hotel room in Siberia—Siberia!—having to watch while someone actually wrote down that the reason we were not taking this beautiful child—and may indeed never have any children—was because, as it turned out, we simply had no warmth in our hearts. The whole thing was beyond obscene.

So here is where—if one buys the idea that marriage is a team effort—I stepped up and, in exchange for that little time-out I'd taken last night while Elizabeth was making all the phone calls, carried the ball a few yards; because though I wouldn't go so far as to say I was feeling *good* at this moment, I had for whatever reason—that second cup of Joe, a taste for the patently absurd, the occasional ability to float outside my body—managed to achieve a queer sort of antihistemic distance from the moment at hand, a kind of benumbed equanimity, drawn principally from the recognition that this—this absolutely ridiculously horrible nightmare of a scene—was, after all, the bed of our making. Part of the reason that last night's decision had been so difficult was because we knew the consequences were going to be ugly, and these were the consequences right here, or the first dose, at any rate. I still couldn't imagine what we'd done to deserve all this—why, at this stage of the game, at this stage of our lives, we found ourselves having to defend and apologize for our inescapable loneliness. Surely there were worse couples in the world some-where. But I could completely see, from the perspective of these three fine, noble, hard-working women sitting before us, that it was incumbent upon them and the system they represented to discourage the kinds of shenanigans we were pulling. For the sake of the children. So there we were. The first slice of doo-doo pie had been served. I picked up my spoon.

"No, no," I sought to clarify, speaking as much to Elizabeth as to the others. "I don't think Polina is meaning to suggest that we actually have 'no warmth in our hearts.' She was simply trying to express that lack of connection that I was talking about . . . "

"To the child," Katya nodded, trying to calm Elizabeth down

Right, I said. See? She understood. I turned to Oksana. "All right, so cross that out too, the bit about having no warmth in our hearts." Oksana looked up at me wearily. What then?

Again, I did the best I could to make it clear, to come up with some translatable phrase that could approximate our experience and at the same time satisfy some distant nameless judge somewhere, and who knows how good a job I did. There was a lot of back and forth, a lot of trying to figure out who exactly *would* be reading this, and why, and would it come up if we tried to adopt again from here or somewhere else; Katya struggling to convey my meaning to Polina, who remained chilly, while Oksana continued to be very patient and obliging, even though the form in her lap was starting to look like a recycled Mad Lib.

And I guess it goes to show the exasperation of the whole effort that I'm not even sure when it happened exactly, but somewhere in there, Oksana looked up from the phone—she'd been on hold nearly the whole time—and said she had just been told that there actually *was* a little boy whose name had just been released, here in Tomsk, a preemie over at the Children's Hospital. Apparently a Russian couple must have just passed on him yesterday or this morning, and we could go see him if we wanted.

Elizabeth asked if they knew anything about him other than that he was preemie?

They shook their heads, I think, but I'm not even sure. I was still preoccupied with the form, and whatever hadn't been crossed out. Elizabeth was still visibly upset. The idea of going and meeting another little boy right then . . . when it has taken all your mettle to back off one diving board, it's not exactly welcome news when someone says, "Hey look, another!"

I pointed at the form again, which was awaiting our signatures. "So if we go and see this boy, is the form still going to be filed?"

It would have to be filed, said Oksana, but no one would see it. Not if we went and wanted this child.

And it wouldn't come back to haunt us? I asked.

No, they said.

You're sure?

No judge would see.

I actually didn't believe this. I suspected that at this point they were willing to tell us anything just to get us the hell out of the room, go see this kid. And I kind of wanted us out of the room too. Elizabeth was even more leery than me, but momentum had taken over. We signed the form. I'm not even sure what it finally said, something about the family not "connecting" with the child. Elizabeth grabbed her purse. I shoved the camera into my jacket pocket, and we all swept out the door.

Out on the street, Polina informed us that she would not be coming with us to the Children's Hospital. She had another appointment, so we said good-bye out there in the open, and all seemed forgiven, I'm not exactly sure why. I think at least she could see that we hadn't made our decision lightly, or maybe it was just that another ray of hope had entered the picture. She wished us luck. We hugged and kissed, and parted ways.

Ivan had chosen to go with the Isuzu today. We all got in—Katya, Oksana, Elizabeth, and me. I was in the middle of the backseat. Elizabeth was to my left, leaned up against the window, drained, scorched, and withered; wearing a halo of tweety birds.

It was probably just as well that we were a little bleary, as I think on some level we both understood that this whole deal—the life we'd been picturing together—now hung in the balance; that if we got to this hospital and met this other boy and had the same horrifyingly nondescript reaction—if we found ourselves looking at each other, wondering what the other was feeling, and was it the same absence we felt in ourselves—and if we then had to turn around and tell these good, kind people for the second time in two days that we don't know, we still don't feel it, well then, perhaps it was time to take a step back and assess. What *were* we doing? What had we been doing? It sure didn't seem likely that we'd be packing up our bags and heading to Moscow—grimy, kind of scary, and nauseating Moscow—just to hop on a*nother* rickety plane bound for some new and unknown region of Russia, a town that couldn't possibly possess the charms of this one, get to know the people there, get taken to *another* orphanage and meet *another* little boy or girl. On what would we be basing our hopes? No, if this didn't work here, then maybe it was time to admit that this whole idea, us being parents, was just a square peg banging against a round hole.

I still wasn't doing too badly mood-wise, though. I was in the throes of a kind of combat-induced delirium. I looked down at Elizabeth, brows high. "You gotta admit, this is livin'. Can't say nothin's happenin' now."

She offered something between a groan and a sigh. We took each other's hand and Ivan wove us through the midday traffic, straight for the sound of the guns.

———

Like most buildings in Tomsk, the Children's Hospital looked closed from the outside. No lights on anywhere. No cars in the lot. But it was definitely hospital-sized, and flat and square and blocky. Ivan drove us around to a side entrance, and Oksana led us in. I was coming to appreciate Oksana more and more. She was quieter than Polina and Katya. She waited to be asked, but her answers were always certain and positive. "This can be done." Really, I could think of no one I'd rather have been following at this moment.

Inside, we ascended another dim flight of stairs that brought us to a long dark hall, banked all along one side by windows, but the day had gone white. She asked us to wait there while she went to see if the coast was clear.

There was a chest-high file cabinet up against the wall, with an baby placed on top and tightly swaddled. All I could see was the face, peeking out at us from under its hat like a little doll. A moment later, a mother emerged from one of the side rooms to retrieve it, and a moment after that Oksana appeared down the hall, waving us to come along. They were ready.

The corridor opened to a larger space and then curled around into an office, with plants and working lamps, a long couch, and all the usual diagrams of uteruses and testicles.

This was the office of Dr. Dobinskaya, the doctor in charge of the ward. Shorter than Dr. Yuliya, with more of a square face, strong features, and cropped, bleached hair with dark roots. She greeted us with the firm grip I'd come to expect from all Russian women, and proceeded to talk us through the child's chart. Katya took notes.

His name was Sergei. I had trouble hearing the last name. Prosenikov? He had been born at thirty weeks. The mother was young, twenty-two. Sergei had been her third pregnancy. There was no information about the father. The mother had basically come in, had the child, and left. No relatives had come to see him since. His birth weight had been three pounds. He had been diagnosed with perinatal encephalopathy (surprise surprise), and that as result of his prematurity, he also suffered anemia, abnormality in his kidney function, heart valve irregularity . . .

I glazed and did some math, but my brain was functioning at about a third-grade level. Thirty weeks? That sounded fairly early, no? Excuse right there. And three pounds, Geez. But how early are we talking about? Pregnancy, nine months. So 9 x 4 = 36 weeks? . . . right? 36 or 54? 36. So 30 weeks means six weeks early.

Six weeks wasn't so bad. Six weeks was doable, and from what I could gather, Dr. Dobinskaya was making it sound like the boy was doing okay. Up to nine pounds now.

The door opened, and there he was, a little bundle on a nurse's arm. Notably smaller than Ilya, who had been sixteen pounds. The nurse handed him to Elizabeth first, a prop for a Christmas pageant, a football wrapped inside a blanket.

I had to round behind her to get a look at his face. He was in a pink cap tied underneath the chin. Cute face. Elfin. Maybe even a little Smurfy. He held his hands up near his chin, rolled into protective fists, but his eyes zapped right onto Elizabeth's. He was small, but there was something very sturdy about him. She said so, and it was true. There was something awfully self-possessed about him, too.

She held him a while. There wasn't as much up and down. He wanted to be close. She rocked him standing, then handed him over to me for a turn. I wanted to cradle him as well, but something about the transfer made him uncomfortable. He started twisting, craning. He reared back trembling, turning red like he might explode. It was a little alarming. I lifted him to my shoulder. He spit up on the towel and it passed.

Could be digestive, said Dr. Dobinskaya. Preemies' intestinal tracts take a while to develop fully.

I made room on the couch and she set him down on his stomach. I removed his bonnet.

Oh, but look at his head. His head was oblong. You could see—from sleeping on one side, and no one being there to turn him.

I took out my camera and began snapping pictures. I figured Dr. Levinson would want to see this. I pointed. "But that changes, right?" The women all nodded. Babies' skulls are like modeling clay, especially preemies'.

Red hair. A high, what some might call "aristocratic," forehead if it were on an adult—the Leslie Howard pattern. Or Prokofiev. He kind of looked like Prokofiev, in fact, that slightly goofy élan. He was trying to push himself up to see—everything, all at once—behind him, above—and for everything he saw, a new expression. He was riveting.

Dr. Dobinskaya excused herself. It was just us, the team and the boy.

I picked him up and held him again. This time he curled right into me. I held him up high on my right shoulder, swaying. He started hiccupping.

Oksana commented something to Katya, with which she agreed. "We were saying, he looks like you."

This was true, too, tribally. The fair coloring. A similarity around the muzzle, though his face was far more acrobatic than mine. With one glance at the window he ran through more perfectly distinct and differentiated emotions than I'll get to in a year. I'd never seen a face so lively, so alive. As his eyes continued to dart about the room, his brows were literally dancing.

"It's funny," I said, a little drunkenly. "I mean, it's kind of silly, I guess, but you know, a big part of the reason we came to Russia is because I've always liked the music so much, and the reason I like the music is Prokofiev. . . . "

They nodded.

"And tell me if I'm crazy, but he kind of looks like him, doesn't he?"

They nodded, obligingly. "And maybe he will have Sergei Sergeievich's talent," said Oksana.

Damn straight, I nodded. I'd looked at his hands already, his fingers. Five each, all present and accounted for, like little star-fish.

Katya was glancing down at his file now. She pulled open the drawer. "Well, and his name," she said, smiling. "His given name is Sergei Sergeievich."

They both laughed. I laughed, too, but they cannot possibly have known how much this meant to me.

I sat down with him. I actually entered into a near full recline. Small as he was, he lay high against my chest, head on my shoulder. I could feel his heart. He could feel mine. He craved warmth, and contact, but he wasn't frail. He was strong, the way you'd have to be to make it from three pounds to nine, alone. He was still hiccupping.

"So ten weeks," said Elizabeth, to them.

Oksana nodded.

Ten weeks what? I thought.

"Early," said Elizabeth.

"Not that many," said Katya.

No, I agreed. "How long is gestation? Gotta be thirty-six weeks, right?"

"Forty," said Elizabeth.

Forty? Pshaw, forty. Forty weeks is ten months. I can do *that* in my head. Pregnancy isn't ten months, is it? Unless you're a whale, or an elephant or something?

But they all seemed to agree, forty weeks was right, give or take.

"Months are more than four weeks." Elizabeth pointed out.

Oh. Right.

Then that *was* ten weeks early. That was a little breathtaking.

He didn't feel ten weeks early. He looked sturdy. You can't be that alive and not be sturdy.

They granted, the starting point of gestation was often inaccurate. Most women count from when they miss their period.

There, I thought, so that's a two-week fudge right there. Still I knew, the bare fact of his prematurity—if we had seen his numbers on a referral back in the safe confines of our apartment in New York, we would have made a paper airplane out it. Three pounds birth weight? That's a glass of milk.

But we weren't back in New York. We were actually holding him, and so yes, fine, that can't be good, missing out on the final two-and-a-half months of gestation, but just to look at him. He was a marvel.

Elizabeth saw it, too, obviously. She must have used the word "fighter" five times, and of course I know one is advised against ascribing too much meaning to the behavior of a three-month-old, especially one who, gestationally speaking, is more like a one-month-old. Just because he looks strong, just because he looks like he could perform a one-man Shakespeare production, that didn't mean he could or will, we knew that.

Still, when I looked into his eyes, the light inside, and all the expression surrounding it—the way his features all curdled into a cry, those amazing brows, and the impish curl at the edges of his mouth—I thought to myself, if this child can grow up to experience even a fraction of the personality, a fraction of the emotion and the life that this face was clearly created to reflect, *I want to be there*. I have to be there. And that's when it hit me, the reason Elizabeth and I had been having such a hard time of it since we'd left New York was that we'd been asking the wrong question. The question wasn't, Does this child belong to us? The question was, Do we belong to him? And the answer was yes.

Yes.

I knew. And I knew what Elizabeth had been talking about the night before when she said that someday we would know why—this was why. This child here. I knew as he nestled down into the cradle of my right arm, we'd got him, and that with all respect to Tim, this little boy was the longest Bomb anyone ever threw.

Elizabeth, less given to audacious mental pronouncement, looked at me—cautious but hopeful. *Do you think?*

I said, "What, do I need to be hit with a sledgehammer?"

No. In fact, I could feel the weight lifting already, but more than the lifting, dissolving, vanishing. I was already experiencing the most mysterious of all human defense mechanisms: the complete inability, once the pain has gone, to remember what it felt like. Even after all that had happened, we felt like the two luckiest, most blessed people on the face of the earth, with that boy now sound asleep on my shoulder.

———

But wait, there was the catch. Oksana and Irena said we had to decide—right there. This was a Friday. The Ministry had us leaving Tomsk tomorrow, which meant we had to file today.

Elizabeth looked at me, and I knew what she was thinking. There were a lot of medical questions, and we still Dr. Levinson on the payroll back in New York, waiting to advise.

Elizabeth turned to Oksana. "There's no way we could extend our stay?"

Oksana shook her head. The Ministry's had our itinerary. We were leaving tomorrow.

"But we couldn't have just a few more hours? Just to try to contact our doctor."

Oksana granted, the papers wouldn't have to be filed until four thirty. It was around two thirty right now. That gave us two hours.

The nurse came to take Sergei back. I handed him over, but this time I didn't want to let him go. The thought of him being returned to his crib, and lying there alone was a fresh new wound in me.

But we were now in a good old-fashioned race against time, and our chances didn't look good. Three p.m. here meant two a.m. back in New York City, and we had to lock in with our decision by four fifteen.

We careened back to the hotel, and all spilled out. Oksana left us there and went to inform the people at the Ministry what was happening. Elizabeth ran upstairs to get all our contact information for Dr. Levinson and another doctor in Moscow whose name we'd been given. I paid for our final night at the hotel, then it was straight back to the State University Internet café, where by now we were old hands. I gave my camera to the girl behind the counter for downloading, we slapped down thirty-three rubles and headed for our computer.

It was a ritually sound but comically pointless exercise. Elizabeth was rifling through all our papers, but Dr. Levinson's notes made fairly clear that she was not to be called at home, so unless the good doctor happened to be surfing the net at three in the morning, there seemed little chance she would get these pictures and meds until tomorrow. She had, however, replied to our last e-mail, the one about Ilya. On reviewing the photos and his meds, she was giving him her highest marks. "All parents should be so lucky."

Ahem. I uploaded the photos of Sergei onto a new e-mail, attached the meds and hit send.

We returned directly to the hotel so that we could sit by the phone, basically. Katya said she would stay nearby. If we got any word, we could call her on her cell.

So we sat and we waited. Elizabeth had an old family friend, a doctor who was living in Turkey, which wasn't so far from our time zone. She tried tracking down his number through her mother, but to no avail. Her mother wasn't home, so we sat and waited some more, and ate our sausage and crackers.

After about half an hour, I spoke up. I said this was absurd because a) we weren't going to hear back from Dr. Levinson in the next forty-five minutes; and b) even if we did, we knew damn well what she was going to say. She was going to say what we'd paid her to say: Don't do this. Ten weeks early, born at three pounds in deepest, darkest Russia? That was way-high risk. That was cliff diving in Acapulco.

"But that's her job," I said. "Her job is basically not to get sued by us."

Elizabeth agreed.

"But she's just going to be looking at a bunch of numbers. We held him. We saw."

"He did seem like a fighter."

"He did. He clearly is."

She thought. ". . . But we're not doctors."

No, we weren't. I couldn't argue with that. She thought some more, her concern deeply etched on her brow. Finally she looked up at me. "But we need to be clear," she said. "He really might have severe medical problems. Are we prepared for that?"

She was asking for the both of us, so I answered for both of us.

"If he's got problems, he's got problems. The question is, do we want to be the ones to help him?"

I looked right back at her. Easy question.

"So we're committing?"

"Yes."

"You want me to call Katya?"

"Yes."

Elizabeth picked up the phone.

Katya was still nearby, as promised. She said she would be right over with the paperwork. I went down to the café to buy some soda.

I was very happy. There was a drinks refrigerator just inside the café door. I got us a Sprite, a Pepsi, and an iced tea. As I paid, I couldn't help overhearing another couple, American. They were having trouble explaining to the women in the café kitchen: they wanted to warm up a bottle of formula. They wanted her to boil a pot of water and put the bottle in. Another man in the café, claiming to speak English, was trying to help, but the whole exchange was chutes and ladders.

"No, honey," the husband said at one point, "that's where you're losing them."

I couldn't help them either, obviously, but I stuck around just because it was great to hear an American accent again, even an exasperated American accent, and because I wanted to introduce myself. I was feeling magnanimous. This was my cigar moment.

Their names were Amy and Burke. Here from D.C. and pretty evidently so—that is, attractive, smart, probably very funny and profoundly secular. They'd just gotten through their court appearance. They had the baby in custody, but it turned out they'd had an experience not so different from ours, turning down their first referral—albeit back in D.C., on video. (I withheld my sniff: "Oh, on video. How heartbreaking.") But Burke said that was the first trip was definitely the hard part. "It's all downhill from here." He pantomimed the hill headed down and I gathered his meaning, even though that phrase has always made me a little nervous. We exchanged e-mails and congratulations. They awaited their formula, and I took my bottles back up to the room.

Katya arrived moments later. Everything had happened so last-minute, she hadn't had time to get a fresh Statement of Intent form. She had a copy of an old filled-in one. We would have to handwrite ours and sign it, that would be fine. Elizabeth's penmanship is a little neater than mine, so she took up the pen, while Katya showed me a book she brought of old photographs of Tomsk; endearingly, she never missed an opportunity to toot the local horn. She flipped through like she was reading to a class of nursery schoolers. ". . . And this is the *pyoly-tyechnical* institute, which we saw . . . And this is the State Theatre." I nodded giddily—"Look, Elizabeth. We were there yesterday, remember? Where we were going to slit our wrists?"

We gave her a copy of my children's book, for her and her daughter, who was thirteen and liked Linkin Park. Katya looked at some of the illustrations. She read a paragraph, nodding. ". . . I understand very well. You are clear."

I said I tried.

We started talking about music then, I think because the form required that we fill in the child's name, the name we intended to give him. We didn't have one yet, so for now we went with Sergei Sergeievich Hansen. Katya revealed that she had studied piano in college. I jumped right in; I'll always talk about music. Who was her favorite? Bach. What Bach did she play? She said the Partitas. What a coincidence, I said, I play a half-assed version of the Sarabande of the First Partita. So who were her favorite players? She mentioned an Israeli she'd seen in concert, but I could tell her scope was limited as an audiophile. By the Russian market? I didn't want to presume, but she'd never heard Glenn Gould. Roslyn Tureck. Not even Richter's Bach, the late-Richter, the sheet-music-reading Richter. Well, we would have to do something about that, I said. I made a mental note: Katya was going to get a major infusion to her personal music library.

We blabbed on thusly until Elizabeth was finished. She signed, I signed, and it was done—a few hours later than expected, and a different boy, albeit, but hey, details details.

Elizabeth was spent. I, who had done a slightly better job sleeping and a much better job eating, was bouncing off the walls. So she would nap. She would find that quiet, dark, peaceful place she hadn't been since our Lufthansa flight. I wanted to go outside. I took the camera and went for a walk.

Really more of a saunter, or a hop. Bobby Van had nothing on me. I eschewed the main way, Lenin Way, choosing instead to head back up the side street so I could get some pictures of those whackadoodle cedar houses with the cross-hatch corners, the doily-like window casings.

Four blocks down I came to one of the parks, divided down the middle by train tracks. On the river side were paths and fountains. The other was a little more woody. I entered to find that the trees (mostly birch, of course) were providing shade and cover for a pretty elaborate amusement park. There was a giant fort under construction. A small roller coaster. *How well they care for themselves here*, I thought, *and their children.* Between the pony rides, the tilt-a-whirls and the women in white slacks, I wondered by what right I was taking this boy away. Maybe when he was nine, we'd bring him back. Buy a summer cottage. I took photos of the fort, the lookout tower. Refrained from immortalizing two teenagers who I think were smoking pot. I crossed back over the tracks and took photos of the pony rides, the fountain. The sun was splashing down. A little boy wearing a beanie was hopping up the terrace steps.

I rounded back for the hotel, took Lenin Way, but I didn't

want to return to the shade of the room just yet. I was too happy, too busy soaking in what had occurred in the last twenty-four hours. The far side of the world, I tell you—the landscape may not look all that dramatic, but I had discovered a valley lower than I thought possible, and a mountain much higher, and I was right up there on top.

Behind the hotel was a little open market, beyond the stand where we'd bought our chicken yesterday. I scoped for fruits I didn't recognize. And tchotchkes. I took a shot of the peasant women with their cups of cedar nuts, and then returned to the room, bounding through the plaster dust and up the stairs.

Elizabeth roused from her slumber, smiling.

"There's a farmer's market!" I said. "You really should see. Fresh fruit!" We'd forgotten there was such a thing. But she still wanted to rest. I asked what I could get her. I felt like we'd been eating gristle and mayonnaise for the last four days.

Whatever looks good, she said. Bananas.

Bananas it is! I bounded back down the hotel stairs and bought bananas, and an orange, and some plums.

Elizabeth was still asleep when I returned. I let her be. God knows she'd earned it. I closed the bedroom door and treated myself to a pretty tasty orange and some Russian TV.

We both called home later that night after dinner. Elizabeth called Anne. I called my parents, got my father this time. I assumed my mother had told him about this morning, that we'd passed on the child we'd come all this way to see, though we didn't know why. I told him we knew why now, we'd met him this afternoon, and we would be adopting him as soon as they let us.

My father understood completely.

Saturday, 7/31—But here's an interesting difference between Elizabeth and me. We returned to Moscow the following day, as scheduled. Once again, we would be spending a night at the enormous and slightly forbidding Ukraina. We'd barely set down our bags when Elizabeth said she wanted to go to the computer center and see if Dr. Levinson had gotten our e-mail from yesterday, the meds and photos of Sergei. She wanted to know what Dr. Levinson thought.

I told her I'd rather sneak up on a donkey and tickle its nuts, because that's about how pleasant I figured the experience would be, and I was right. When Elizabeth returned from the computer center (no, I did not go), she reported that Dr. Levinson had indeed received our e-mail, and offered that in her professional opinion she could not advise our proceeding with the adoption of this child.

So off we hobbled to dinner, but managed to shake off the blow by dessert. That is what we'd paid her for, after all.

CHAPTER FOURTEEN

THE WAIT

I think from the moment we learned that Russian adoptions require two trips, Elizabeth had been dreading this part maybe most of all, the interim; dreading it as I had been dreading that nine-hour return flight with the wailing new baby, but much more, of course. And that was before we knew that our child—the child we had committed to, at any rate—had been born ten weeks early, and was as such likely to suffer developmental delays and any number of other conditions, whose lasting effects could be greatly diminished the sooner we got him home and could start giving him the care and attention he needed.

Both Polina and Ronni had said to expect a wait of four to eight weeks. It turned out to be twelve. Three months. Not that I was all that surprised. We'd been warned that once you get into August, the Russians start going on vacation. Also, the Tomsk 400th Birthday celebration was scheduled for the first week of September, so that was sure to slow things up. After that was anyone's guess, but I'd resigned myself to the Rule of the Private Contractor: Multiply all best estimates by three.

But knowing why we had to wait didn't make the waiting any easier. We could try to go about our days as usual, but the fact remained there was a little boy, a very little boy, over there on the far side of the earth, lying in a crib, all his synapses waiting for something to fire at, but with no one there to hold him, roll him, mold his little head back into shape. Did he understand that he had met his parents, that that somewhat drained-looking couple who came to see him that one day and held him briefly, they thought he was a miracle, and they'd vowed to return? That if he could just hold on, stick it out, they would be there as fast as they could, to take him home and put him in his own crib, with his own stuffed animals and blanket, and that he would never, ever, ever be alone again, or without a home? Did he know?

It would have been nice to think so—that somewhere in us all there is an instinct for knowing when we're being thought of—but good Catholic upbringing notwithstanding, this was slender consolation. And as the days passed into weeks, the whole thing began to seem a little unreal. We didn't tell a lot of people, but we did tell some—the nearest and dearest—and in the honing of the story, it did begin to seem a little like a fairy tale. It was hard to believe it was true, maybe because it wasn't—yet. We didn't have him.

Elizabeth was hounding Ronni on the phone, but to no avail. We wondered, only half-kidding, could we hire Katya's daughter to go in and hold him for an hour a day? But we didn't even know if he was still at the Children's Hospital or whether he had been moved to an orphanage. We were basically cut off.

No question this was all much harder on Elizabeth. Being a teacher, she is used to things happening when they're supposed to. When they don't, she reads trouble, and her mothering instinct was starting to kick in strong.

I was doing a little better. I am pretty used to things not happening when they're supposed to, and I spend half my life waiting for people to call who don't. So I did manage to get back to work. I set up some meetings with potential editors for the John book. Kept mulling the outline, kept tooling with the adaptation, and otherwise distracted myself in the usual ways.

The wheels had come off for the Mets, but the Red Sox were making a run at the Yankees. Hurricanes were shredding Florida. Iraq was turning into a disaster area, but it looked like Bush was going to win re-election anyway, or re-whatever-you-want-to-call-it; in our nation's ongoing struggle between the forces of *Hee Haw* and *Laugh-In*, *Hee Haw* was still in ascendance, remarkably.

More notably, the last week of August—the fourth week of our wait—two Russian commercial airplanes crashed in separate but nearly simultaneous incidents, the work of Chechen Black Widows.

One week later, on September 1—which the Russian people celebrate nationwide as the first day of school—a group of armed rebels took over a school in the town of Beslan. Two days later over three hundred people were dead; one hundred eighty-six of them children.

Did these last three incidents touch us more than they would have? Definitely. That image of the parents sending their children into school with balloons in their hands—Elizabeth and I could see the smiles on their faces much more clearly now. And when the mothers saw those same balloons go rising unaccountably into the air, the first sign that something had gone terribly wrong, we could see the anguish on their faces, too, and feel at least a fraction of the horror.

But did I detect any portent in it, or personal cause for concern? Not really. My reaction was oddly politicized, in fact, perhaps because of the looming election and the sinking feeling I was getting. It wasn't so hard to imagine a world in which an incident like this would be greeted with a meaningful demonstration of solidarity, or might further galvanize the community of civilized people. One didn't have to be an idealist to think that such a thing might be possible. As it was, the disjointed quality of our response and the response of other nations—signing books of condolence—only served to underscore how fractured the world had become, again. No one could speak with moral authority. No one possessed it anymore. No one could lead, because no one would follow. It was, to me, further proof of how much our "leaders" benefit by the sheer scope of their corruption; the fact that their misdeeds are all judged in context of one another; that we can so easily be distracted from this lie here by that one over there, or the supposed flaws and treason of their critics. If just once we measured them against the standard of what else might have been, the magnitude of their failure and treachery would finally be clear. . . .

Oh, well.

On the truly domestic front, Elizabeth and I did what we could to get ready. We made an album of photos of our apartment: the yawning crib, the park, and our families, all to show the judge in court the world awaiting our son. I had an old tweed suit of my uncle's tailored, bought new shoes. We finally got news about Ilya: Another couple had come to see him, and would be adopting him. So that was a relief, if not too big a surprise.

We looked at the photos of Sergei on the computer

We stopped looking at the photos of Sergei on the computer.

We chose his name. I'd liked "Sergei," obviously, but we didn't want his teachers asking him about it every year on the first day of school. So after a fair amount of deliberation, sounding out the various possibilities and permutations, and printing them out in a variety of handsome fonts, we finally decided to call him what he was, and to recognize his birth name by sticking it in the middle and using a Latinate form, Sergius, in honor of one of Russia's patron saints, St. Sergius of Radonezh, a man of the wilderness in the mold of John. I hadn't known until we did a little research, but one of my favorite paintings by Nicholas Roerich was of St. Sergius. *The Builder*, it was called: bold lines and bolder colors set forth a bearded man in a hilly, wooded landscape blanketed in snow. He is bending over with an axe, chopping wood either to warm a nearby cabin, or to finish building it, and he is all alone, but for the silent, peaceful witness of a brown bear.

In mid-September we finally got a medical update on Sergei, but the information was minimal and not good: His weight was still low—off the charts, even for preemies; and the head circumference wasn't too great either.

The evening after we received the news, we wandered around our neighborhood looking for somewhere to eat. We settled on Ruby Foo's, I think just because they boasted lots of specialty drinks. I had two Singapore Slings. That's the only time I've ever done that, drank to dull myself.

It worked okay, I guess. But I didn't shut down completely. The truth is, throughout that whole stretch, what got me through—more than my distraction with politics, or baseball, or even my work—was the confidence I had in him, or whatever that was inside of him. I'd felt it when I held Sergei, something awfully powerful had gotten him from where he started—no bigger than a hand, with lungs the size of lima beans—to where we found him, that hilarious, squirming, nine-pound bolt of life. Whatever that was, I trusted it to sustain him until we got back there.

I trusted that, because that was all I could do.

October 12, first week of the playoffs, we got our dates. We were to leave for Moscow in three days.

CHAPTER FIFTEEN

THE VERDICT

As uncomfortable as the wait had been, there's no question that the second trip to Tomsk was, in prospect at least, much less nerve-racking than the first. We knew where we were going this time. We knew the people we were going to see there, and the place; maybe three months colder, but the same.

Even so, Burke, my D.C. friend's, assurance that "it was all downhill from here" lingered in my mind as the perfectly ambiguous oracle. Certain elements of suspense definitely remained, after all. There was the court appearance; there was the return flight, if all went well; and of course there was Sergei's health.

We flew Swissair this time, via Zurich, and I guess our anxiety was showing early. The moment we touched down in Moscow, Elizabeth got hit with a pretty bad headache. We'd booked a room in an airport hotel to spare ourselves the ride into the city—we were due to fly to Tomsk first thing the following morning—but we'd barely set down our luggage when Giorgi called to inform us that there had been a scheduling mix-up and that if we wanted to see Sergei tomorrow, we should probably leave for Tomsk tonight, like right away.

There didn't seem much choice, so wearily we re-hoisted all our bags and shuttled back to the airport. I practically had a hernia, our luggage was so heavy this go-round—what with all the extra clothes we'd brought for warmth, and for Sergei, and gifts for the orphanage. Elizabeth barely made it out of the hotel van before vomiting on the curb of the terminal.

We then had to grease the palm of an airport official just to get on the plane. He promised first class, delivered bulkhead, which was fine, though probably inadvisable since it planted us right in front of the emergency exits and we spoke no Russian. No matter. The exits were blocked by passenger baggage anyway.

Four hours later, we arrived in Tomsk, six a.m. local time; this now after two straight red-eyes, back to back. Katya and Ivan were there to pick us up. Old friends—but much more, of course—war buddies—and all in good spirits, or as good as could be expected after Beslan. Katya admitted, that had muted the birthday celebration, and one could sense the tears that had been shed, but life was moving on. We picked up Polina on the way into town, and made straight for another old friend, the Hotel Siber—same room, even. While Ivan stayed in the car listening to the news, Polina and Katya joined us upstairs to go over our schedule.

They reported all good things about Sergei. He had been moved from the Children's Hospital #1 to the regional orphanage, not the same as the one Ilya had been in. She said we could see him this morning. The pre-trial hearing was set for tomorrow, then the actual adoption hearing was two days after that.

"And this is where the famous writer will prepare something beautiful to say." A speech in court, she meant. That was the first I'd heard anything about a speech, but they said it would be a good idea, and the truth is, if you call me "the famous writer," you can pretty much get me to do anything. I'll mow your lawn.

We spent the rest of that first meeting basically chatting, catching up. We showed them the photo album we'd made of our extended families and where we lived, all so the judge could see what sort of life we were offering Sergei. We'd even included a map of Manhattan to show how close to the park we lived. Polina had never been to New York, but she showed a remarkable familiarity with the highlights. We pointed to where the Metropolitan Museum was, and Lincoln Center.

"And Trump Tower?" she asked.

Right there, I pointed.

"And Saks Fifth Avenue?"

The regional orphanage was on the other side of town from the municipal, standing out among what looked like old warehouses and vacant chain-linked lots. It was a bigger facility than the municipal. It looked like a small hospital—symmetrical with a recessed entrance, and painted white.

The biggest difference on the inside was the presence of the other children. At the municipal orphanage, we hadn't been allowed to see any babies other than Ilya. Here, the moment we entered, there was a small procession of them coming downstairs together—toddlers, all climbing down in the variety of styles you might expect from a dozen two-year-olds: butt-first; sitting, one step at a time; those who could were holding hands. They were all in caps with earflaps, and all wearing the same slightly flared snow pants patterned in the same native hieroglyphs. More poignantly, there was apparently a case of chicken pox working its way through the orphanage, and Russian calamine is blue, so in addition to the Little Bear hats and matching snow pants, their faces were spackled with constellations of coral blue.

They were still very cute, though. Some clearly had challenges yet to overcome, were suffering from one syndrome or another, but most were perfectly healthy and bright, and heartbreaking, their story was so clear. No doubt they'd been diagnosed with some condition when they were infants, something dire enough to frighten off any prospective parents, but now they were clearly fine, just two or three years older.

Some smiled and pointed when they saw us. They understood who we were, and why we were there, but they also seemed to know it wasn't for them. People like us, we come for the littlest ones.

As the nurses led them out into the cold crisp air, we were called into the office of the head of the orphanage—another woman, a little older than either Dr. Yuliya or Dr. Dobinskaya, but again, exuding professionalism, care, and competence. She had prepared a statement about Sergei's overall progress, but she had trouble getting through it—I'm guessing Elizabeth interrupted her five times with questions. She answered each patiently, over the top of her reading glasses, but asked again if she could simply be allowed to finish. The moral was he was doing well, the overall diagnosis being what they called first-degree prematurity.

"But so that's like burns?" I asked. "First degree is better than third?"

Yes, she nodded, the dainty chains of her reading glasses gently seconding the motion.

There was some discussion of the birth mother as well, more than I was comfortable with. Katya was taking notes, but I tuned out a little, not because I was afraid of what I might hear or because I didn't want to humanize her too much—or not *just* that—but the whole conversation struck me as being a little too conjectural. Apparently they hadn't been able to track her down, so she was either out of the region or still "indigent." They'd used that same word back in July, but what did that mean? No address? Elizabeth and I had already discussed this: No address for a thirty-year-old would have meant something, but twenty-two? That could just mean you're sleeping on your friend's couch, in which case half the twenty-year-olds I've known were indigent. I guess the novelist in me comes out at such moments—not because I think I know the story. Quite the opposite, because I know there could be a million explanations for anything—including leaving the child you just gave birth to at a hospital—so unless I see some evidence, I tend to withhold judgment. All I really cared to know right then was about this young woman's heart—the one beating in her chest, I mean—and her liver, whether there was cancer in her family, or strokes, or schizophrenia. And this they could not tell me. The personal stuff, we could sit and guess, but we'd end up learning more about ourselves than her.

In any event, the conversation was cut short by the entrance of the star of the show, Sergei Sergeievich.

He did look well. Rounder. His hair was darker. His skin was smoother, clearer. No chicken pox, thank God; if he sprouted so much as a single pock, we would not be able to leave the country with him. His head still had a flat spot on the back, but it was better.

We took him straight up to the second floor. There was an open area with doors all around, but near the top of the stairs was a window and a pair of oversized easy chairs set beneath a mural of Snow White and the Seven Dwarves. That's where we had our reunion. We'd been there for about thirty seconds when Sergei let fly with a pretty ample jet of spit-up, right on the shoulder of my blue-green sweater. And not innocent baby spit-up, either. Something about the formula they were feeding the kids gave this spew an awfully vomitous quality, and I don't care how happy you are to see someone, vomit fumes wafting off your shoulder will take you out of your game. Elizabeth did most of the doting after that, but my impression was still one of great relief. That spark that we'd been trusting in, the force that had gotten him through his earliest days, still seemed to be prevailing; that, and the care of all the nurses and doctors, who deserve roses forever.

He was also, however, still showing clear effects of prematurity and orphanage living. His hands were still up around his chin. He was doing most of his reaching with his tongue, which was understandable—bottles and pacifiers had likely been his only real stimulus for the last three months—but it was a habit we would be trying to break; it made him look a little like a gangster's henchman. His stamina was limited. He was more passive than I remembered him being, even more so during our afternoon visit with him. We went right back after a quick lunch, and he seemed a little spacey. He had no interest in the plastic keys we'd brought. His eyes still darted around, but a little frantically, and he wasn't making much noise. Also, toward the end of both sessions, he started turning his head back and forth, as if he were hearing bells on opposite sides of the room; it seemed a little manic.

This concerned me. I didn't say so to Elizabeth at dinner, but the curator for the museum of my life should definitely try to get his hands on the bed in room 318 of the Hotel Siber. Heavy hast my head lain on that pillow. I was wide awake at five a.m., staring at the ceiling, confronting the possible as the inevitable, that our apparent moment of grace and inspiration back in July might just have been another trick. Something was wrong with him.

It turned out Elizabeth was awake as well, feeling the same dread; no second thoughts, of course. We had accounted for this. We were his parents and we were there to help him, but we were definitely girding ourselves.

When we got to the orphanage that morning—entering to a chorus of toddlers upstairs, clapping their hands and singing to a piano accompaniment—we asked to speak the head of the orphanage again.

She saw us right away and was very reassuring. She said all the behaviors we'd been noting were typical side-effects of orphanage living. The manic rocking of the head was a self-soothing mechanism.

Of course, of course, we nodded. We'd just wanted to be sure. We thanked her, and when Sergei was brought out to us that morning, it was as if he'd sensed our concern as well. We went up to the Snow White mural again, and he was much more lively and alert, pushing himself up on his hands, smiling, baby-talking. The same child we'd met three months ago—hilarious and profoundly familiar.

Maybe the best indication of how much better we were feeling was that Elizabeth decided that afternoon to get her hair done before the pre-trial hearing. In a Russian salon. Without Katya there to translate.

Now that's balls, I thought.

Especially since Elizabeth had been getting more and more anxious about our court appearances. Even back during the first trip in July, she'd been pestering Polina and Katya with questions about it. How often did judges refuse couples?

Katya had been pretty clear. "Very rare."

"How rare?"

"Almost never."

(*Oh, great*, I thought.)

"Almost? How often?"

Katya tried to remember. Maybe one time she could think of.

"Why?" asked Elizabeth. "What was the judge's reasoning?"

Katya squinted, trying to remember. "I don't think there was a reason. I think the judge just didn't like them."

Ah, fuck. Not that the story bothered me—I instantly pictured Joel and Hedda Nussbaum and sided with the judge—but I could see the seed had been planted in Elizabeth's mind, and I watched it grow over the course of the next three months: this one measly incident, dragged with a crowbar from Katya's memory, the clear moral of which was that these things *almost never happen*, magically blossomed into indisputable proof that these things *do* happen, and that we had better take every possible precaution to look like June and Ward Cleaver when we walk into that courtroom because there was no telling what these Russian judges were basing their decisions on. Sometimes they just didn't like the looks of you. Katya said so.

Anyway, Elizabeth's hair looked okay when she got back. The stylist had tucked it under. Perhaps not my favorite of the retro looks we were going for. I might have gone with more of Laura Petrie curl-out, but it definitely could have been worse.

The courthouse where our hearing took place was located farther inland and upland from the river, just beyond an Orthodox church with a giant bell. We were a little early, so Ivan gave us a pep talk in the car, through Katya. It was the first time he'd really offered any advice to us, and so it carried extra weight. Leaning around in his seat, gesturing freely with his massive hands, he told us that what the judge would be looking for—more than reassurances about our health or finances—was conviction. If we simply conveyed a firm intention—that this is what we wanted, and this is what we were going to do—that would carry the day.

I didn't doubt he was correct. Conviction is all anyone anywhere is looking for.

This was just the pre-trial hearing, though, and was, as billed, a formality. Highlight, the judge. A woman. Tall, very slender and angular, with high Slavic cheekbones, and spiky blond hair—I'd have guessed mid-forties—but tough. No-nonsense. In fact, I'm not sure she even looked at us—just shuffled through the paperwork as she ran down the questions—names, birthdays, boom, done.

As soon as we were back outside, I told Katya that if all went well at Friday's hearing, I'd let her in on some colorful English phrases for a woman like that.

First legal hurdle cleared, Elizabeth and I decided to keep it simple that evening: ate dinner at an underground English-style pub whose walls were lined with gold records from the 1980s—notably, Scorpions. We went over the speeches we intended to make in court: I'd be handling all the touchy-feely stuff; Elizabeth would explain in more practical terms how we intended to care for the child.

We turned in early, Elizabeth earlier than I. I read and watched some TV. Our friends the Tomsk soccer team were playing. I couldn't locate the captain, though, and got caught up in another show, a nightly half-hour news report devoted exclusively to local traffic accidents: cop car pulls up; checks out the damage; someone complains; cop car pulls out. This happened about five times until the final segment, which featured two old women in long coats and headscarves imploring a homeless man to come out from under a park bench, it was too cold to stay outside. The old man wouldn't budge.

————

We continued seeing Sergei, of course, for morning and afternoon sessions, though by now we'd graduated from the plush chairs in front of the Snow White mural to the actual playroom. The older children we still saw occasionally, a blue-spotted, bow-legged procession of toddlers in various stages of dress, sometimes all in underpants, headed in for naptime. They seemed to be on a different rotation than Sergei.

Our visits now were coinciding with those of a young Russian woman, single, who was adopting a baby girl just Sergei's age.

Arina was to be her name, after Pushkin's nurse, and she tended to wear a matching pink hat and pajamas for the occasion. I couldn't tell how fetching Sergei found it. There was a lot to look at: rocking horses, balls, masks, and a wall-length mirror, and mats of course—chicken pox sponges. We laid down towels and kept our fingers crossed, and watched him continue to bloom before our eyes. Each time we saw him it seemed he had a new trick, like a new petal opening, but only to reveal the spirit we'd known was there from the first.

And he was getting to know us, too. At the end of every session, instead of the nurses coming for him, we would bring him back downstairs to the room where they kept the infants. There were four or five cribs in the room we saw, each one with two bouncy chairs inside. The children were all slotted in and fixed with pacifiers, helpless to do much more than turn their heads as the white-smocked nurses shuffled by with either towels or white pots of mush. As we handed Sergei over one morning, the nurse who seemed to be most in charge of him commented that we must be spoiling him upstairs. He'd been so content before, and quiet. Now he cried when he was left alone.

———

The morning of the trial, two social workers came to the orphanage to observe us with him. One had exceptionally long, honey-colored hair; to the knee, I'm guessing, though she kept it up in an elaborate braid. The other was her senior. I don't remember her hair, but they were both very kind, and approving. They could see we were perfectly comfortable with Sergei by now. For the better part of the visit we talked about Saint Sergius and the Roerich painting.

We had our outfits all picked out, of course, for the main event that afternoon. I wore my uncle's old suit—newly tailored, but still with an early-1960s cut, boxy, conservative with slightly pegged legs. A solid, wheat-colored tie. Elizabeth: pink cashmere top, brown jacket, tweed skirt. Attractive, but without attracting too much attention. Her sister Anne had helped her pick it out.

When we got to the courthouse, we were made to wait a while, first outside in the hallway, and then in the courtroom, which was hot. They were pumping the heaters, so we opened some windows. Katya was visibly nervous. I wasn't entirely sure why. She said she was worried about the petition to change Sergei's name— that we might not have gotten it in on time. This didn't strike me as that big a deal. Whatever happened here, we could fix later, but it was actually good that she was so anxious. It made Elizabeth and me feel like the calm ones, and I did feel calm.

There was an actual prison cell right there in the courtroom, built right into the benches—maybe ten feet long, seven feet high. When I looked at it, I imagined it was filled with all our friends and family, all the lawyers and doctors we'd used over the years, and nurses and counselors and limo drivers, everyone who'd helped contribute to this moment—all scrunched up together in the cell as if they were on bleachers, with pennants and popcorn and soda. They were all very excited.

Finally the principals arrived: the prosecuting attorney, the two social workers, a court reporter, and last but not least, Her Royal Highness of Iceland.

As soon as the proceedings began, I realized why Katya had been so nervous. She had a *lot* of translating to do. It was coming from all sides, very fast, and most of it in legalese. There was a great deal of repetition about the child's situation. The social workers both testified—about us and about how little was known about the biological mother.

It finally came our turn to speak. The crowd in the cell fell silent. I went first, and tried to keep it slow, for Katya's sake. Keep the bites small.

I actually thought about including a transcript of the entire speech here for your benefit, but in looking over it, I have to say, it's really quite long. It began:

> *I am told that Russian television runs a soap opera called Santa Barbara. Well, right next to Santa Barbara is a little town called Carpinteria. This is where my mother grew up. . . .*

I kid you not. I don't know why, but I was possessed by the soul of David Copperfield. Basically I stood up there and delivered them the first nine chapters of this book—courtship (check); desire to have kids (check), IVF woes (check), switching over to adoption (check). I even got into the bit about always loving Russia because of Prokofiev. I can only say in my defense that part of the strategy was to go a little long. Polina had said, the more Elizabeth and I talked, the fewer questions they were going to ask, and I think I did at least succeed at that. By the time I rounded the bend and was headed for home, the room was pretty well tuckered out.

So let me just pick it up there . . .

. . . And it is this same fascination and sense of connection that finally caused my wife and I, in considering the homeland of our adopted child, to turn to Russia with a great sense of hopefulness, excitement, and humility.

But we chose not only for ourselves, not simply because it would give me the chance to clasp hands with a people who've enchanted me for so long, but most of all for the sake of the child.

Make no mistake, Elizabeth and I will make a home for him. He will enjoy the full embrace of our families. He will have an abundance of aunts and uncles and cousins to play with; ranches and orchards and beaches and parks; doors he can knock on that will always open for him and take him in, homes and hearths where he can sit and (be warmed) loved and accepted no matter what. He will be proud to be a Hansen. He will be proud to be a Woodworth.

But we also know that some day he will want to know about the place he comes from originally. We do not know when he will ask or why, but we want to be sure that when he does, he under-stands that his native land is a place we love too, and care about deeply, and that if he wants our help in finding it, we will be there for him with full and open hearts, as we intend to be there for him in all things.

To her credit, the judge was not remotely taken in by my overt cultural pandering. Her first comment after I'd finished and we'd given Katya a glass of water, she pointed out that my affinity for Prokofiev wasn't going to help much if and when the child began to develop any of the medical complications that often attended prematurity, and had I taken such possibilities into account?

Score one for the judge.

Fortunately, Elizabeth had prepped me for this one three months earlier, back in the hotel room just before we committed to Sergei. I gave the same reply, that if the child was prone to certain conditions, he would suffer them with us or without us. The question was whether we wanted to be the ones to take care of him. The answer was yes.

Score one for Professor Peepermeister.

The judge tested our resolve in one more, even slightly more curious, way. Following Elizabeth's less voluble account of how we planned to raise the child, the judge asked her if we had thought at all about the fact that he probably came from a different social class than we did.

I have to say, I hadn't seen this one coming. And to this day I'm not even sure if she was preying on the perceived classism of American society, the perceptible classism of Professor Peepermeister over there; or merely reflecting the entrenched classism of her own culture, wrought as it was—for several centuries, at least—by lords and serfs. I really don't know, but I did at that moment realize how American I am—i.e., how thoroughly indoctrinated by all those Prince and the Pauper stories we like to tell—because I almost didn't even understand the question. Elizabeth, either. She answered that we didn't consider Sergei to be of *any* class.

"He is a baby," she said, with just the right note of confusion.

Score one for Teach.

But let me not leave you in any further suspense. The prosecuting attorney had no further questions. It was Friday—getaway day. The judge excused herself briefly, for a drumroll. This was it. Elizabeth and I clasped hands. The judge returned about thirty seconds later. Crowd in the pen all held their breath as the she read the verdict aloud, and Katya translated:

All petitions granted.

We were parents. We had a son.

And Theo was his name-o.

———

That evening, the sky with a shudder of relief shook down the season's first snow, but home was still a few days away. Between now and then was a fair amount of paperwork, and a lot of thanking to do.

Our visits with Theo *(-dore,* if you're wondering) were fewer than we'd have liked. Just the mornings now. When not with him, we were being shuttled around Tomsk by some combination of Ivan, Oksana, Polina, and Katya—doing what had to be done: picking up his birth certificate, his medical forms, his visa papers. The day after the trial, we drove back to the courthouse to pick up the verdict. We brought flowers, as a perishable (i.e., legal) token of thanks to the judge. We got to see her in her chambers, and I actually think you may have seen this scene on TV a few dozen times: mysterious motorcyclist removes mirror-visored helmet to reveal . . .

. . . what a lovely woman she was, not just physically striking, in jeans and a white linen shirt, but warm, and gracious, and funny. I'd brought a book for her as well, and signed it. She said her husband would love it; he loves historical fiction.

Then it was back to the car, we had more gifts to see to, more papers to sign and collect. It struck me as we shuttled from place to place that one of the unintended inspirations of this whole process was how vividly it recalls infancy—for the parents, I mean: you're constantly being shoved into the backseats of strange cars; you never quite know where you're going. You can't understand what anyone is saying. You don't really know what food you're eating, and you always kind of feel like you're about to vomit. It's a nice touch, just before you're about to become a parent, getting a crash-course reminder of what it means to be a baby.

For some balance, we decided to treat ourselves to a dinner at one of Tomsk's two finest restaurants, the one by the river where Chekhov was said to have eaten once. The woodcuts on the wall could have been by a number of different members of my family. The drapes were a William Morris pattern. Odd.

Otherwise, it was all car, all the time. There was one day we didn't even see Theo at all. We just drove around Tomsk buying gifts. There was apparently a pretty strict protocol to be observed, so we deferred to Polina, contributing our opinions only when called upon. That day we bought:

- a bathing set for the regional social worker;
- a bathing set for the orphanage social worker;
- a bottle of Kenzo perfume for the judge (to be given through a friend, hence legal);
- another bottle of Kenzo and a bottle Martini and Rossi for the head of the orphanage;

- a jar of Platinum instant coffee for the orphanage workers;
- two chocolate cakes for the orphanage workers (and a money donation as well to the orphanage as a whole);
- one jar of Platinum instant coffee for the folks at the visa office;
- one signed copy of *Monsters of St. Helena* (my most recent) for the judge's husband, a reader apparently;
- one signed copy of *Caesar's Antlers* for the Moscow judge who was so helpful in expediting our trial dates.

When our spree was finished, we had a little party in our suite, except for Ivan, who remained in the car. We had havarti cheese, cedar nuts, pears, and white wine. Katya toasted, then Oksana—toasts to Theo, giving thanks for what was utmost here, that he had found a home in which he would be safe, and cared for, and thrive. Polina quoted an old Russian aphorism: no good without bad; that is, no fortune comes but from misfortune. I raised my glass and echoed the sentiment. Theo may have got off to a rough start in this world, but he'd been blessed ever since. How many children could say they had four guardian angels?

Then Elizabeth and I gave them the gifts we'd brought.

For Katya: one Native American dream catcher; a butterfly bag from the Museum of Natural History; a Juilliard shirt for her daughter; and three Bach piano concertos played by Gould (1, 4, and 5).

For Oksana: one Native American dream catcher; a matching blue hat and scarf; the Byron Janis recording of Prokofiev's Third, performed in Moscow in 1955.

For Polina: one Native American dream catcher; a William Morris scarf from the Metropolitan Museum collection; late Richter playing Bach live, French suites as well as the "Capriccio on the Departure of His Most Beloved Brother."

For Ivan: a bottle of Cointreau, some chocolate, and air filter for the Jeep Grand Cherokee, as requested.

Then Katya and Elizabeth and I went off to a concert up the street, an organ recital featuring more Bach.

———

The Wednesday following our court appearance, and the day before we were to leave, Elizabeth and I finally went to pick up Theo at the orphanage and take him away for good. We'd brought a little snow suit for him, and handed it over to one of the nurses. We didn't see any of the other children that day. We just waited in the lobby with Katya, under the watchful eye of the aged nurse who manned the desk.

When they finally brought him out, he was nearly lost inside the snow suit, it was so big. Just his face poked out of the collar, but he looked up at the nurse as she handed him over to us, and he smiled a smile of thanks more sweet and filling than all the chocolate cake in Siberia, I'm sure. We put him in a green wool cap that Elizabeth's mother had knitted for him. The nurses all waved good-bye. I grabbed our bags and Elizabeth carried him outside into the scattered snow drifts. Her smile was blazing.

As Ivan and Katya drove us back to the hotel, Ivan commented. "So you'll be back in the spring for a sister."

I laughed. *Could be,* I thought. Not spring, though. It would take a while to figure out how many years this had either added to or subtracted from my life.

That evening, Elizabeth fed Theo a bottle of formula by the window of our room, a radiant blue of twilight and snow. A while later I rocked him to sleep for the first time as my son, and set him down in the little playpen the hotel supplied. He lay on his back, arms wide open, utterly trusting, utterly peaceful

We left the following morning at dawn. Fittingly, the winter arrived full-force to see us on our way. Though the sky behind was still dark, we stepped outside the Hotel Siber into a white-out blizzard. The people of Tomsk likely would not see the ground again until May.

Ivan said not to worry. The plane would leave on time, and I didn't doubt it. No carrier called Siberian Air can be all that squeamish about a little snow. So we all crammed into the Jeep, all nestled in our parka down, and Ivan drove us back up that long tree-lined road to the airport. The windshield looked like bad reception on a TV.

I'd mentioned that car-accident show to Ivan the previous day, and he had revealed to me—somewhat boastfully—not only did he *not* use chains in the winter, he didn't even change his tires. And yet even as we skidded and skiied along the snowy road on Ivan's bald Firestones, unable to see more than six feet in front of us, I didn't feel all that nervous. Not even with Theo in my lap, eyes wide. I felt alive. I felt the same as I had all those years ago when Nick and I had pedaled through the black from the train station, guided by nothing but the white dashes on the pavement and the occasionally passing car, knowing that a fallen limb or little rut could well have taken us out, but also feeling sure it wouldn't, not if we found the right speed.

The snow was still coming down heavily when we got to the airport, but Ivan was right. The terminal was packed with passengers, all shuffling toward the gate, and we could see three or four other couples in the crowd, Americans, with their translators and their new sons and daughters—a sight both humbling and comforting. We weren't the only ones, and they each had their own harrowing tales to tell, no doubt, starting way back when they first fell in love, and leading them all right here, to this very same, very happy, very tired spot.

We said good-bye to Ivan and Katya at the gate, the time had come. We hadn't many words at our disposal, and what words would have sufficed? These people, and their colleagues back in town, probably just rising now, drinking their morning brew, they had given us life, and hope, and all the things we'd started to doubt we'd ever have again, all bundled up in a light blue snow suit much too big for him. Ivan looked down at Theo in Elizabeth's arms and took his thanks from that, the certain knowledge of the boundless swarm of love that boy would live in from now on.

Finally though, we turned our backs for one last time, telling ourselves we would see them again, this wasn't the last time; we would send pictures, and notes. And we would think of them every day, and we have. Every day.

But now it was time to be just the three of us in two small seats, finally headed home. The morning light had come. As soon as the workman ploughed away the snow, our aged little plane lumbered down the runway and heaved itself into the air, and the lift pulled Theo's eyelids closed again. He drifted off to sleep, and I looked out the window, as Tomsk, the river, the rolling hills of Siberia, and all the mountains and valleys of our Antipodes disappeared beneath the clouds.

EPILOGUE

We spent two days in Moscow before returning to New York. We had business there as well—Theo had a required medical exam, and a visa to pick up. We decided to indulge ourselves and stayed at the four-star, and very Westernized, Sheraton Palace; definitely the best thousand bucks I ever spent.

The day of our arrival also happened to be the day of the deciding game in the Red Sox/Yanks ALCS. The Red Sox had climbed back from an 0-3 deficit to force a game seven. I couldn't find anywhere in Moscow that was televising the game—not at four a.m., anyway, so I made several calls to the States and had a combination of my brother, my mother, and Nick call me in the room with inning-by-inning updates, all in exchange for a word or two with Theo, provided he was awake. It was a very gratifying return; and even more so when we finally got back to our apartment in the city and flipped on the Red Sox/Cardinals World Series games to see all those banners in the crowd: "Thank you, Theo! For Breaking 'the Curse'"[2]

Oh, and the flight was fine, by the way. Except for the part right at the beginning when we were taking our seats and Theo was hungry and crying and I was trying to open the formula carton with a pair of baby nail clippers. That was kind of a drag, and a mess, but otherwise, smooth sailing. Those six-month-olds, they really don't know the difference between a plane ride and a rainy day.

---

2   Theo Epstein presumably, the Red Sox GM.

About a year after all that, I attended a small reunion dinner—four old friends who half a lifetime ago traveled through Europe together for about six weeks one summer. Twenty years later, it was—happily, if not all that romantically—the meeting of four devoted fathers. The intervening twenty years had seen their normal share of striving and discovery, unexpected triumphs, and bygone aspirations. But regrets, that was the question. The senior fathers at the table all agreed, no. Parenthood had fixed all that. Whatever had happened in their lives, personally or professionally, it had brought them their children (all girls, oddly), and that gift was so precious, they would not take back a single breath, for fear it might disturb the path that led them to their daughters.

I'm aware that I began this with a vow not to succumb to such reasoning. Just because one is happy at the present moment, that can't mean you never made a mistake, never wasted time, or that *all* the pain was worth it. I know I wrote that, I know that sounds right, and I know that now I'm not so sure. It seems to me there's an element to the equation that never occurred to me before, even though it's pretty obvious when you think about it, and that is that the roads we take do more than merely lead us to our destinations; they prepare us too.

I think of those two voices that kept battling for our attention as Elizabeth and I worked our way through the adoption process—the one that said be *open*; the one that said be *sure*—and how they were right there with us in Tomsk, speaking in our ears as our moment of truth drew near. It strikes me now that we relied on both, and both in the extreme; that as fated as what happened to us those two days may seem to us now—first meeting Ilya at the orphanage, then Theo at the hospital—it would not have unfolded that way but for all the stubbornness we could muster, and all the openness as well. And I guess I don't believe that either of those reserves would have been there, or been so deep, if it hadn't been for all those years leading up, including all the heart-break and the anger and the sorrow. They're not just what got us to Tomsk, and they are what got us through Tomsk, too. They are what let us find our son, and in the end, that really is all that matters.

ACKNOWLEDGMENTS

Finally, my sincerest thanks to all of those who have helped to bring this book into being (and who will be named): the partial list includes Sam Hansen; Hope Grey; my agent, Sarah Chalfant, for her ongoing commitment; Pat Johnston; John Brody, for resurrecting the manuscript from its drawer; and all the rest of the people at *Best Life* magazine, but especially Steven Perrine, and Bob Love. Likewise the corps and core at Modern Times—Angela Polidoro, Meredith Quinn, Chris Krogermeier, Beth Tarson, Marina Padakis, Joanna Williams, and Tara Long, but most of all, Leigh Haber, for not forgetting that this story was out there, and for believing it had the chance to do some good.